Advance Praise

....

"*Live Your Life, Not Your Diagnosis* is powerful and empowering. Hanson shares a fresh, brand new, systematic guide to reframing one's perspective and living with a difficult diagnosis. *Live Your Life, Not Your Diagnosis* inspires turning weakness into strength, conveyed in compelling ideas with vivid stories to which everyone can relate. The personal steps equip readers with explicit ways to draw on their inner courage and trust of self to do things they never thought possible with the hand dealt.

"Hanson's book is not solely about looking multiple sclerosis in the 'face' and embracing a more abundant life. The nuggets of wisdom are a rich gold mine—elegantly laying out a realizable plan that is applicable to any diagnosis, helping those who have suffered a major loss, whether from journeying through death, divorce, a broken relationship, or other major life setbacks, such as career or life disappointments. I will be recommending *Live Your Life, Not Your Diagnosis* widely to all my patients when dealing with a diagnosis or setback!"

SANDRA BOND CHAPMAN, PhD
Founder and Chief Director, Center for BrainHealth,
Distinguished University Professor, author of *Make Your Brain Smarter*"

T0163667

"Andrea Hanson has written a spectacular book. If you have been diagnosed with MS, you've struck gold by finding it. It's a guiding arm around you as you navigate what to do. But even without a specific diagnosis of multiple sclerosis, you will benefit from Andrea's wisdom. The lessons she teaches and the exercises she provides will help anyone who is struggling with any type of medical diagnosis or challenge. I read this book in one sitting and marveled at the wisdom Andrea offers in a very humble and casual way. It's an easy and enjoyable read that could truly change your life if you apply what you learn. I highly recommend you do."

BROOKE CASTILLO
Master Certified Coach and Founder of
The Life Coach School

"So many books written about MS are cathartic for the writer but overwhelming for the reader. It is refreshing to have a book that fosters hope and promotes self-healing. This book will work best for those who are willing to do the accompanying exercises; doing these exercises will increase self-awareness and self-connection—two very powerful tools that the author advocates strongly for, and that I believe are essential perquisites for self-healing. Ms. Wildenthal Hanson does not claim she is an expert on MS; instead, she does something much better: She encourages the reader to become his or her own expert. I believe this book is an excellent resource for those newly diagnosed with MS who are looking for ways to be proactive… and ways to find hope."

CINZIA LEVALDS, PHD
Licensed Psychologist

"I can't wait to tell our patients about Andrea's *Live Your Life, Not Your Diagnosis*! I'm so thrilled Andrea has written this book to encourage people diagnosed with multiple sclerosis or any chronic illness. It is a true guide on how to listen to our bodies, connect to them, nurture ourselves, and understand the power of our mindset. I think people will relate to her stories—the good, bad, and funny. There are several exercises for people to do through the book, keeping the reader engaged and active in their health care. I think this is a must-read for anyone diagnosed with multiple sclerosis. Love it!"

KATHERINE TREADAWAY
LCSW, MSCIR, CRND

Live Your Life, Not Your Diagnosis

LIVE YOUR
LIFE

*.not*Your.
Diagnosis

How to *Manage Stress* and *Live Well*
with *Your New Health* Condition

ANDREA WILDENTHAL HANSON

NEW YORK

LONDON • NASHVILLE • MELBOURNE • VANCOUVER

Live Your Life, Not Your Diagnosis

How to Manage Stress and Live Well with Your New Health Condition

Published in New York, New York, by Morgan James Publishing. Morgan James is a trademark of Morgan James, LLC. www.MorganJamesPublishing.com

The Morgan James Speakers Group can bring authors to your live event. For more information or to book an event visit The Morgan James Speakers Group at www.TheMorganJamesSpeakersGroup.com.

ISBN 9781683507956 paperback
ISBN 9781683507963 eBook
Library of Congress Control Number: 2017915752

Cover Design by:
Rachel Lopez
www.r2cdesign.com

Interior Design by:
Chris Treccani
www.3dogcreative.net

Editing
Grace Kerina

Author's photo
Courtesy of Angela Weedon Photography
www.weedonphoto.com

Author's logo
Created by Steph Calvert
www.stephcalvertart.com

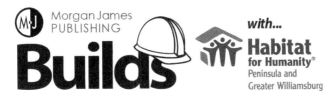

In an effort to support local communities, raise awareness and funds, Morgan James Publishing donates a percentage of all book sales for the life of each book to Habitat for Humanity Peninsula and Greater Williamsburg.

Get involved today! Visit
www.MorganJamesBuilds.com

Disclaimer

· ·

Dedication

....

*This book is dedicated to the millions of people
impacted by multiple sclerosis.
Whether you have it or love someone who does.
Whether you research it, treat it, lobby or volunteer for it.
We are all in this together.*

Table of Contents

....

Foreword

....

By Elliot M Frohman, MD, PhD, FAAN, FANA
Director, Multiple Sclerosis and Neuroimmunology Center
For Advanced Care and Discovery
The Dell Medical School at the University of Texas at Austin

Having served as the author's neurologist, diagnosing her soon after I arrived at UT Southwestern Medical Center in 1995 (from Johns Hopkins Hospital; where I completed residency and fellowship training), to organize the institution's first comprehensive and multidisciplinary treatment, education, and research Center for multiple sclerosis and related neuro-immunological conditions, I was not at all surprised when I first learned of Andrea's writing initiative; to construct "Live Your Life, Not Your Diagnosis".

Over the 30 years of my career in medicine, I have come to recognize the veracity of my own mentor's proclamations; that "while patients do not teach of everything about medicine, without a doubt, they teach us the most important things. And if you pay very close attention, each individual patient has distinctive elements to share about their experience, with having an unpredictable, chronic, neurological disorder such as multiple sclerosis (MS)."

A core principle of this highly approachable, honest, compassionate, and hopeful compendium of 'PEARLS AND PITFALLS' focused upon living 'well' with MS, is Andrea's extraordinary 'in-sights', as a true 'insider' as an MS patient, to understand that a fundamental frame of mind, is characterized by the statement; "I may have MS, but MS will never have me!!!" She is among the most positive thinking patients I have known over the course of my career.

To be clear, crisis, tragedy, alteration or abolished neurologic capabilities, do not represent sequences of life's most challenging events, from which great 'characters' are built and refined. Alternately, I have always believed that the most formidably challenging facets that must be confronted by the journey we must all take, do NOT build character (sure we can and should learn things from such events), but instead they 'expose character'.

As underscored throughout this delightful book, Hanson understands that for those who alternatively believe that the disease process "has the upper hand in controlling my life", are at a dangerous predisposition for actualizing the self-fulfilling prophesies that can be scripted as:

1. *I can't*
2. *I'd love to, but what's the sense, MS will just knock me down and over; it's the boss!!!*
3. *What's the point of taking my medicines adherently, when they are not cures, and that each and every one of them have serious side*

effects, in conjunction with exorbitant pricing of the MS disease modifying therapies; are they really worth it?

4. *I just know that I'm doomed, and my doctor did not feel strongly about my starting and taking MS medicines; I could just tell.*

5. *What's the use, it's all about the drug companies making profits for shareholders, not delivering life sustaining, and quality of life improving agents for me, and others like me.*

6. *Even if I take the MS medicines, I just know I'll get worse anyway; I always do.*

7. *My doctor, and his physician extenders (nurse practitioners and physician assistants) neglect to ask me, what I consider to be the most important questions, that I would like to have answers to; or at least a hypothetical explanation to my most important questions.*

8. *My care team never asks me about those most sensitive questions that revolve around bowel, bladder, and sexual dysfunction associated with my disease process.*

9. *My doctor and nurse practitioner both emphasized the importance of escalating medicines gradually over time, for management of symptoms, until one of three things occurs; a) the medicine works b) we have escalated the dose multiple increments, without any corresponding benefits c) or, there is the emergence of intolerance or toxicity. Nevertheless, I took the introductory dose of the medicine for two weeks, and noted not a single tangible benefit, so rather of advancing the dose as instructed, I instead decided to stop the treatment; it was not for me.*

10. *What's the point of any intervention for this horrible neurological disorder, ultimately it will 'win the battle', rob me of my life's most important personal and professional goals, and all notwithstanding my working diligently and unrelentingly over time.*

All 10 of the above, are in essence powerful indictments upon negative thinking (which like the placebo effect; 'works'; so does too negative thinking, in the opposite direction; a phenomenon referred to as the 'nocebo' effect.

Having defined the distinctive dichotomy between negative (nocebo driving) and positive (placebo driving) patients, such a stratification can levy some of the most important consequences that are fundamentally germane to 'doing MS well'; while never ever allowing this disorder to remove the winds out of your sails, and then attempt to collapse your sails altogether.

With the nocebo/placebo dichotomy now defined, the author proceeds to underscore a landscape of potential areas that patients can volitionally decide greater control and influence over every phase of their lives; including the refusal to give up, and give in. Perhaps not surprisingly, MS patients who are highly stratified to the nocebo (negative) zone of thinking, are much more likely to exhibit reduced adherence with respect to both the utilization of medication (addressing the disease course as well as the disease related symptoms), starting and maintaining a regular exercise program, learning about and adopting principles of healthy eating, and in reduced adherence with performing surveillance laboratory studies and imaging studies. Such nocebo patients might simply say; "what's the point, none of this is going to work for me; I'm allergic to everything; nothing I do agrees with my body; exercise is problematic as I'm tired before I start (as MS patients are like batteries, with the exception of starting out after a recharge (i.e. sleep in this context) with only a fraction of the battery/energy capacity, when compared to normal, healthy, matched control subjects).

A highly salient message that courses through the entirety of 'Live Your Life, Not Your Diagnosis' is that there are in fact many facets to living well with MS, that do in fact exert control over the disposition of the individual's disease course, and ultimately upon their quality of life.

The most important of these is our ability to learn about the disorder that afflicts an individual MS patient and their family. Equipped with such knowledge, patients and families alike can become highly informed, and more effective members of the therapeutic alliance; after all, the MS patient is the most important member of the MS continuity of care team. While the above points emphasize an extremely common constellation of sentiments, it remains the fiduciary responsibility of not just the treating physician, but all members of the care team (including the patient and their family and friends) to ensure that everyone shares a common goal, while equally importantly is the pathway and process by which we can eventually arrive at our target destination; to live a life to the most, and one with an emphasis upon quality of that life.

As a patient with MS, and perhaps the most exuberant and positive 'spirit' I've encountered in my 30-year career, Andrea, too, was not immune to the kind of thinking that can result in a preoccupation with the question; "why me?" and woe is me…and what does it matter anyway, as I have nothing that I can do to change what is going to happen to me (particularly after innumerable and strategically diverse treatment interventions, she continued to exhibit evidence of ongoing disease activity).

Not surprisingly, many patients in similar circumstances, would have made the declaration of treatment failure, and by extension translate this 'failure to benefit' to generalize this one experience to all subsequent interventions; in some cases so strenuously steadfast to this principle (albeit completely erroneous), that the patient deprives her or himself to the next treatment strategy; perhaps even the one that may just be the one to exact remission of the MS disease process, with potential concomitant dividends in the form of 1) exacting remission 2) mitigating symptoms 3) Facilitating the initiation of a more predictable disease course 4) Improved reparative mechanisms that we now know can be associated with improved neurologic capabilities; even the reversibility of deficits, and signs of central nervous system derangements abolished.

'Live Your Life, Not Your Diagnosis' is perhaps the most beautifully architected 'primer' on the subject of multiple sclerosis that I have read to date. It's completely accessible, avoids the very common and distracting digression into areas of information and technical science, which from the outset, was NOT the objective for this book. Instead, I would designate 'Live Your Life, Not Your Diagnosis' as a quintessentially authentic, fair and balanced treatise on 'MS' and how to 'do it well'.

The author is NOT among those MS patients who have had the extraordinary blessing of following an extremely benign course of MS. NO; Andrea is one of those MS patients who have been the recipient of the most 'shock and awe' exacerbations, thereby requiring acute interventions.

As a patient, the author has long-recognized the importance of 1) knowing her mind and her body 2) understanding the effect of the medicine being utilized for MS, and its likely corresponding mechanisms of action, along with the most important treatment related side effects.

Herein, this authority on 'having MS', shares with the reader her experiences upon coming to the 'fork'; systematically analyzing her options, but in the end, decisively 'taking it'. Over the years, Andrea has seen much darkness, but throughout she never quit believing, hoping, and searching; for what? For light and for love. Not just for others, but for herself. This journey that she has 'taken', has validated her self-esteem, confidence, and correspondingly reduced her fears and 'anticipated' negative prophesies. Instead, she has found her way to the place she has so desperately sought since the inception of this disease. A place where she can be confident that even when one treatment and regimen fails to produce the desired outcomes, new options and alternatives will take its place.

Rather than being right, this is a life primer, the principal thrust of which is fundamentally about 'getting it right'. There is a huge difference between the two vantage points and objectives, and without hesitation, Andrea has succeeded to showcase and illuminate those life principles that are easily attained, and do not require long odysseys to distant lands or super specialized clinics. Why not? Because all along, the destination where light, love, peace, and tranquility can be found, is not at all far away; how could it be? For all along, it's been with us; 'INSIDE' us; just as this highly salient 'Guide' will confirm. For those who are willing to journey 'inside', and upon arrival at the place where looking is imperative, those capable and willing to 'see', will find the most incredible gift; if of course willing; it's the gift we give to ourselves. Once we have accepted this gift, we are all equipped to harness the most powerful force in the Universe; LOVE.

While finding yourself through each of our personal journeys is a blessing beyond quantification; there is yet another level of force and of love in this life. In essence, no matter the gift nor its magnitude, the joy, happiness, and satisfaction we receive from those gifts bestowed upon us (by others and by ourselves), all shall be eclipsed by those things we do or give to others. In this sense, Andrea Wildenthal Hanson has brought something truly quintessential to the reader (whether in some way attached to MS or not)…the primer is all about what Voltaire's Candide (1759) espoused on the great mission in this life; but before all, "but first to cultivate our garden". To first get on with the everyday tasks of life, and not be overly concerned with matters beyond our control, unless they are in fact within our control. The author here does something very important; she clearly takes the reader beyond the mundane tasks of everyday life, and instead utilizes a new optic from which the reader can 'see' ahead and into the future (even as soon as today or tomorrow); this optic is called hope and light; which together form the scaffolding upon which the impossible morphs into the possible; and as stated in

Mark 9:23 of the new testament; "all things are possible, if you will only believe."

'Live Your Life, Not Your Diagnosis', if anything, is in fact a roadmap and compass toward that place inside each of us; the place from which we can journey to places long held to be impossible to reach. According to Hanson; not so fast; until you've been on the road I have traveled. One not exclusively mine; indeed, the one I hope to show you, and even take you along it with me. Touché!!!

Introduction

....

Are You With Me?

I was sitting up in my hospital bed, dazed after a long day of being whisked from one doctor to the next. My new MS specialist had just left the room after displaying a large group of MRI films on a gigantic light board. He'd shown my parents and me the bright white spots displayed on the films and said simply, "These are bad." Those "bad" bright spots were everywhere on my brain.

I will never forget his words to me: "You're on fire. There is no doubt that you have multiple sclerosis."

Earlier that morning, I'd carefully driven myself to the ophthalmologist's office because, over the previous few days, I'd slowly become almost completely blind in one eye. Earlier that week, I had coincidentally (and accidentally) poked myself in that eye, and I thought

I had a detached retina as a result. With my nonexistent knowledge of the eyeball's anatomy, a detached retina seemed like a logical possibility. I drove to the hospital for my appointment with my new ophthalmologist, certain I'd get it fixed.

After peering into my eye a few times and seeming a bit confused, my new ophthalmologist called in another specialist. I was escorted down the hall to my next new doctor, who was a neuro-ophthalmologist. He took his turn peering into my eye, but this time there was no confusion. He informed me I had optic neuritis. I waited to hear the fix. Antibiotics? Bed rest? I was ready to wear an eye patch for a week if absolutely necessary. But no, that wasn't the next move. What happened next is that the neuro-ophthalmologist called in yet *another* doctor.

Mere hours later, I sat in my hospital bed, dazed by the events that had transpired that day. It had all happened so fast. I'd been sitting in a regular doctor's office only a few hours ago, consulting with the kind of doctor regular people see about regular people's problems that are pretty quickly fixable.

But now I was in a parallel universe.

One with specialists, pictures of my brain displayed on the wall, and people with very, very serious faces.

I wanted to go home.

My Backpack

After everyone else left for the night, my dad sat next to me on the bed. I was so scared I felt knocked over, like someone had punched me in the stomach and left me on the ground. I wanted Dad to make it better. I have never seen him so upset. Compassionate and determined, he looked me in the eyes and said, "This doesn't stop you. You can still do everything you want to do. This is just another brick in your backpack."

Almost immediately, this new diagnosis made sense to me. It may be heavy, and I'll carry it for life, but MS was only another brick in a backpack containing the bricks I was already carrying. Other bricks represented other circumstances in my life, like the graduate program I was powering through, and my grief about someone I had recently lost. With only that shift in perspective, MS no longer seemed as big and overwhelming.

I was 22 years old when I had that talk with my dad in the hospital. What he said that night helped me form a perspective of MS that has served me well, and will serve me well for life. Over 15 years later, it's still fresh in my mind.

We each have a backpack filled with bricks. Those bricks are the things that weigh heavy on us—at least at first. A brick might be a diagnosis, a debt of some kind, or a grief. Sometimes we get to take a brick out of the backpack, toss it aside, and leave it behind. Some bricks will stay with us forever. No bricks are better or worse than the others. But they're ours to carry.

On that first night of my new diagnosis, thinking about what my Dad said, I clearly saw how everyone is in this life together, each of us carrying our own backpack.

And I knew, right down to my toes, that I would be ok carrying mine.

A World of No

As I lay there hooked up to my IV, various professionals came through to educate me and hold my hand. Some of them, like my MS specialist, were forthcoming about my situation. I felt an immediate bond with him. Other professionals who paraded through my room were not so helpful. I dubbed them the "MS Welcome Wagon." My memory of them is fuzzier. At one point I remember talking with two ladies—although it may have only been one (I also had double vision at the time). However many of them there were, I'm sure their intentions were good. But their message to me about MS was summed up in a big pile of "You can't do that anymore."

Hot Showers? "You can't do that anymore."

Stressing out? "You can't do that anymore."

Pushing yourself and working too hard? "Nope. Can't do that anymore."

Going outside in August? "This is Texas, my dear. You definitely can't do that anymore."

As this "education" about what I could "no longer do" was imparted to me, I thought about the brick in my backpack. My natural tendency to buck the rules bubbled up inside of me. My inner rebel, the one who had created so much trouble for me as a teenager, finally stepped forward and found her purpose. *What do you mean I can't do that? Who do you think you are?* I lay in the hospital and every time I heard someone tell me about something I couldn't do, I thought, *That's not true.*

Every time someone told me I would have to be careful, I thought, *That doesn't apply to me.* Whenever they told me I wouldn't be able to do something anymore, I'd nod while replying to them in my head with, *You don't even know me, so how could you know that for sure?*

I watched as some health professionals put a label on me. I was no longer *Andrea Wildenthal.* I was now *MS.* And because I was now MS, a whole bunch of things now applied to me by inference—no questions asked, no discussion about who I was as a person, no asking if I had experienced any of those symptoms before. None of that seemed to matter to them. Their perspective seemed to be that I didn't understand myself anymore since I'd had the MS diagnosis. Now other people believed they should tell me who I was and how I was going to feel.

Nope, that didn't sit well with my inner rebel *at all.*

MS Is Not My Story

Slowly, over those few days I was in the hospital, I changed. But not in the way all those people wanted me to change. I didn't start planning to slow down and stay away from all things heated. But I did go from stunned and dazed to becoming a little clearer about who I was (or at least who I wasn't). For one thing, I knew the new brick of my MS diagnosis represented a whole new world I had to carry with me, learn about, and manage. For another thing, I knew I could deal with an extra brick. It was just a brick. It was something I could decide for myself how to handle.

Fueled by my 22-year-old inner rebel, and probably also the massive doses of steroids given to me for three days straight, I decided my MS would never define me. I didn't need people who didn't know me to say what was ok for me. I would find out for myself what worked and what didn't, thankyouverymuch.

Somehow, I knew in my deepest well of truths that my vision would come back to 100 percent (and it did). I also knew my MS doctor would find a way to stabilize my condition (and he did). But the thing I knew most of all was also the biggest truth of all.

I knew MS would never be my story.

MS is a part of my story, yes. But it's not how I define myself. It's not the measuring stick I use to rate how I feel every day. It's not my go-to cause when I feel icky. To be honest, some days I don't think of it much at all. And that has nothing to do with what's going on with my MS symptoms. It has everything to do with how I perceive them.

Life changes because life changes. I've learned that I can look at these changes in one of two ways: Situations happen to me that make me change, or I create change because of the situations around me.

I didn't know it at the time, but I decided in that hospital room that I would be the one creating the change. I would deliberately recalibrate according to what felt right for me.

My decision was that I was in charge, not my MS, and so it was up to me to find out how to deal with it in a way that was right and best—for me.

Your View, Your Choice

I wish I could say it was only smooth sailing from then on. I wish, just this once, I could honestly tell you a triumphant *I made the decision and never looked back* type of story. But I can't, because it's not the truth. Such big decisions or changes rarely seem to be simple, linear, or easily resolved. Growth is usually not a straight line to freedom, and anyone who says otherwise is probably covering up a big part of his or her story.

MS is a very individual disease. Everyone's symptoms unfold differently. Because of that, I can't tell you what to do about the way MS shows up in your body and life. What I will do instead is guide you through the creation of a plan that works for you. There is a personalized combination of therapies that will help you. I've laid out a program in this book to make it easier for you to find that unique combination that suits you best.

There is a way for you to ease your stress about hardships and changes in life. There is a way for you to feel better about your new circumstances.

If you have a diagnosis other than MS, or even no diagnosis at all, these concepts can work for you, too. The way to freedom isn't through focusing on the disease. The way to freedom is through focusing on the human that happens to have the disease.

Throughout this book, I share what I've learned that has made all the difference for me and my MS. I've laid out the chapters in the order that I discovered each layer of therapies or strategies that helped me. By finding things that worked and then going on to find more, I've built a combination of elements that works for me personally. You can do this too, so that each time you add a layer, it joins the existing layers and creates something new and better, something that grows organically to help you in a very personal and original way.

Some of the things I'll discuss in this book are tactics I learned about and did that instantly lifted a weight off my shoulders. Others are lessons I learned while kicking and screaming. The most transformative thing I've learned on this journey is that how we look at our health is crucial. It's the most important layer of all.

You can blame your health problems, you can blame something you think you did to cause them, and you can blame people for looking at you differently. Or you can use your diagnosis as fuel for living a better life than you did before.

Yes, that's possible.

There's a difference between letting a diagnosis run your life and running your life that happens to include a diagnosis.

I know which one I choose.

Are you with me?

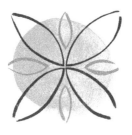

....

Chapter 1

....

Creating Something New

My hunch is that you want to feel in control of your new situation. A diagnosis was handed to you without your permission, and you want to feel confident that you're doing the right things to help yourself as much as possible.

But what you really want is your old life back. You want life to be like it was before your doctor said, "You have _____."

Although being diagnosed may leave you shell-shocked for a while, I bet you're also ready to actively do something to help your prognosis. You wouldn't be reading this book if you weren't. But what can you do *specifically* to help *your* health? You've come to the right place. Over the course of this book, you will find your answer to that question.

It's important to note that I learned what I did because I have MS. You may also have MS. Or you may have another diagnosis, or even something doctors can't diagnose at all. Everything here can help you. If you don't have MS, insert your own diagnosis when I talk about MS. Know that you are included here. You can use the information, the worksheets and the tips in your own way in order to manage stress and live well with your diagnosis, too. We are all in this together – no mater what our bodies are doing.

You're Not Alone

A new diagnosis is scary. Within the five seconds it takes your doctor to speak the sentence telling you the news, everything changes. You now have a new number-one priority, one that shifts everything else down the line. That project at work isn't even a blip on your radar anymore. And your future, once crystal clear, is now a haze.

When I was diagnosed with MS, I felt like I was staring down the barrel of a whole new life, one I hadn't asked for, certainly didn't want, and hadn't even known existed until that day. But I knew I wanted to get through that huge change. I had to. I was not willing to put my life on hold. So I began to take action, which is where a lot of people with a new diagnosis start.

One of the first things I did when I was diagnosed was get a ton of facts. You may be accumulating a lot of information right now about what your diagnosis is and what your diagnosis means for you. When we're faced with a big change, it's normal to want to know everything about it. Your doctor is by far the best source of factual information that applies to you, because they know you and your situation and can give you information that's specifically pertinent. I received all of my information from my MS specialist at first.

But there are also sources like the Internet, pamphlets, professional organizations, research, and other patients' accounts of what life is like for them. This information can seem like an avalanche and feel completely overwhelming. It's hard to know what to make of everything and to be sure of what's true.

You want your MS to go away. You want MS not to impact your life. You want to simply *do* something that you know will help. But what does helping your MS look like? Taking medication? Exercising? Going gluten-free? What should you do and how often should you do it? And will any of it really work? How can you avoid wasting time on all the wrong things?

We dive into action because it feels good to start doing something. Maybe we start with a few things and then aren't sure if they're working. We listen to the experts. We read testimonials from people saying a certain therapy cured their MS, so maybe we start there. We're not sure that's enough, so we try something else. Managing what we "can" and "can't" do or eat or think now that we have MS can consume our lives. And the changes we choose to implement are often quite drastic. At the end of the day, we still feel like we're grasping at answers. And graspy is not a fabulous feeling.

Feeling uncertain and frustrated is actually a good thing. It comes from being passionate about taking action when the answers we need haven't fully formed. If you're feeling this way, it means you've already started moving forward.

The good news is that MS is now better understood than ever before. According to Healthline.com, an estimated 200 people per week are diagnosed with MS in the United States alone. Worldwide, there are over 2.4 million people living with MS, most of whom will not become severely disabled. There are currently 17 approved MS drug therapies to try, if you choose to, with even more in various stages of testing for FDA approval. People are receiving diagnoses earlier because doctors are better informed. We are moving in the right direction.

MS is not a death sentence. But, unfortunately, there's not a cure yet either. So it's up to us to find the right treatments for ourselves.

Getting a Head Start

An underlying theme of the program outlined in this book is how to feel confident in whatever therapy you're trying. In fact, a very important part of choosing a therapy is not about *what* you choose. No matter what the therapy is—traditional medication, exercise, diet changes, stress management, or a combination of all those and more—how you *feel* about your choices is extremely important for producing helpful results.

You may have heard of the placebo effect. It occurs when people take a sugar pill, believing it's a medication, and their symptoms diminish. Their belief affects their symptoms. The efficacy rate of a placebo can be as high as 50 percent.

The same is true in reverse. Someone can take a powerful drug and believe it's a fake—and even though they have real medicine in their system, they don't get the full effect of the drug.

We create our own personal placebo effect when we believe in the effectiveness of the therapies we choose. What you expect to happen influences what actually happens. Believing in what you're doing gives you a head start before you even fully form your plan.

Let's Talk Statistics for a Moment

I'm not going to tell you what symptoms you have an 80 percent chance of developing. I'm not even going to tell you what MS symptoms are common. I don't believe statistics like those are useful, for a number of reasons.

Statistics change when there's new input data. MS research moves fast. Every year, there are new drugs and new revelations about how MS works. Doctors are constantly updating how they treat MS. With those changes come more new data, and more new statistics.

Hearing those statistics can create expectations within us that something will go wrong for us in the future. That expectation can harm us more than it helps, because it can shape our thoughts and beliefs, and thus our reality. This happens even if we aren't fully aware that we internalized the belief that a negative event is on the horizon.

We may think statistics are helpful, but the data behind them may have nothing to do with us individually. Interviewers and scientists aren't basing their statistics on people exactly like you. They talk to and work with people who have MS, but those people are still different from you. They're living in different circumstances, getting different treatments, having different symptoms, dealing with MS at different ages, stages, and with potentially other conditions present as well. An MS diagnosis may be the only thing you have in common with the people who were polled or studied in a way that led to any given statistic. Additionally, very often a similar medical or social study will yield entirely different statistics about the same population. So it is hard to know what external source to believe.

I'm not saying this to discredit science. I believe very much in the power of data. What I'm saying is the way in which we internalize data is crucial. We must remain aware of if we're seeing data as proof of something scary or horrible happening to us, or if we're seeing it as simply information.

What You Expect is What You Get

A primary focus of this book is the benefits to be gained from connecting with yourself and becoming fully aware of what is true for you personally. Attention to statistics and trends can distract our attention away from ourselves, skewing the conversations we have with other people and with ourselves about our MS. That's because of something called *expectancy theory*. Robert Rosenthal is known as one of the first researchers to examine expectancy theory. He conducted a famous experiment with teachers and elementary school children. Researchers gave children ordinary IQ tests, but told the teachers that the kids had received special IQ tests that predicted which children would experience a rapid increase in IQ as they grew. The tests actually predicted no such thing. The results of the study showed that the children who were "predicted" to have a rapid increase in IQ actually did. Those who weren't "predicted" to have an increase in IQ didn't.

Researchers found that when teachers thought a child had a high IQ score, they changed their interactions with that child slightly. The teachers gave those children a little more time to ask questions, a bit more attention overall, more praise, and more feedback. They expected those children to have a boost in IQ, and a boost was indeed reflected in the subsequent performance of those students.

What this study and the placebo effect both show is the incredible power of expectations. What others expect to see in us changes how they interact with us, even though they often don't do it consciously. These changes in how people react to us can then manifest an unwanted result—if we're not paying attention. Similarly, what we expect to get from any therapy we try can alter its effectiveness.

Our expectations of ourselves are no different. This is known as *self-fulfilling prophecy*: What you expect is what you get.

How do our interactions with ourselves change when we expect a symptom to occur? Do we live on, trusting the future, not worrying? Or do we focus on the symptom, watch for it, and eventually begin to see that symptom emerge?

What if we expect to develop MS fatigue, for example, because we read that there's a high probability we will? What about when we're talking with a doctor or nurse who expects us to develop certain symptoms because that's what they typically see every day in their clinic? As people living with MS, we're surrounded by other people's expectations of how it will affect our well being, and what will happen to us. We can either put our belief in what other people think will develop in time, or we can be aware that their expectations are not the same as our own reality.

Better Expectations

What if you had an expectation of health? What if you truly believed that you could handle your MS, and you fully expected your current course of therapy to work? What if you altered the way you acted toward yourself as a result? What if you became more nurturing toward yourself? Or would you rather turn away from this whole issue and let someone else tell you what your expectations should be?

Choosing an expectation of health is up to you.

It's important to know that being diagnosed with MS doesn't take that choice away from you.

Almost immediately after I was diagnosed with MS in 2000, I knew I wanted to expect health. That doesn't mean I somehow fail if I have a relapse or I don't achieve perfect health. It does set up a habit of expecting well-being, and that habit can take me a long way. I still approach everything—from my workouts to my medication—with the belief that they are helping me manage my MS, and helping me be well in general. Sometimes an aspect of my plan for managing my MS falters or I have a bad reaction. Because I expect wellness, I expect those bad reactions to diminish. I expect to learn from those experiences. Because I'm focused on what's happening with my body, I'm able to notice subtle changes and I know pretty quickly if something needs attention or is improving.

Expecting Health

This book is designed around expecting health. I'll show you exactly how you can connect with yourself and with what's happening right now. I'll show you how to let go of the expectation that something bad will happen.

That's why I'm not going to load you up with statistics. I won't tell you the intricacies of how some studies show that MS can hurt some people. I'm not going to tell you to look for symptoms you may never develop. I'm not even going to tell you much about the symptoms I've experienced, because I don't think that information is relevant.

I will never, ever say that you will "suffer" from this disease, because I don't believe people with MS suffer from having MS. I believe the suffering comes from other things, which are generally within our power to change.

I'll show you how to find true, unyielding hope within yourself, however much you may be questioning its presence or strength right now. I'll direct you toward actions you can take to help yourself around your MS. I'll tell you stories about myself and stories about clients I've worked with who have MS. I'll emphasize the stories that illustrate ways of not only overcoming challenges, but also getting through to the other side of them even stronger. I'll show you how you can start making powerful decisions right away.

I'm also going to share about two important pieces of information I believe are missing from a lot of wellness plans: the questions of "Why?" and "How?" These questions are often overlooked because people want to hurry up and move on to taking action. But *why* we do something and *how* we do it have huge influences over our self-connection and the strength of our motivation.

Most importantly, I'll show you how to create a plan that gets you feeling confident and in control, because that's what we're ultimately after.

This book is full of information I've learned from more than 15 years of having MS and five years of being a life coach. I've created a program to help people who are newly diagnosed with MS craft a master plan of action tailored to their own needs.

Without a doubt, there are things you can do right now to help you manage your MS. This book is a guide to what has helped and continues to help me and the other people who have gone through the program. This book and the program are here for you, to help you figure out what to do to take control of your own MS management.

Are You Ready?

When you combine a strong belief in whatever you're trying out, a deep connection with yourself, and an awareness of what your body is feeling, you create a powerful way to harness expectations and move toward health. You take control of what you want to do and how you want to do it. You stop grasping at answers because they sound like they might work, and then not being sure if they made a difference. Instead you find out whether they actually work for you. You skillfully put together teams of professionals to assist you in your quest for health. You acknowledge that no decision is made in vain, because you're willing to learn and adjust as you go. You can become your own expert and courageously create your own life with MS.

As a life coach, I focus on change. This book can help you create huge changes in your life—changes that *you* control. But it can only happen if you participate. I suggest keeping a journal handy while reading the book and doing the exercises, which have been designed to help you gain a deeper understanding of each concept.

DOWNLOAD YOUR OWN FREE WORKSHEETS.
Go to *www.AndreaHansonCoaching.com/BookSheets* to get full worksheets of all the exercises in this book.

For the past two years, I've specialized in working with women who have diagnoses like MS. No matter who I'm coaching, if they have the belief that they will create positive change and succeed in obtaining their goal, success happens.

Carol Dweck, researcher and author of *Mindset: The New Psychology of Success*, writes about how our beliefs about ourselves shape our results. She says, "The view you adopt for yourself profoundly affects the way you lead your life."

What view do you want to adopt for yourself? Will you adopt a view that expects you to have little say about your MS? Or will you choose a view of expecting to continue to learn and to contribute valuable input to your MS management?

Who do you want to be as a person living with MS?

I've asked a lot of people that question. Their answers vary from "Calm" to "Courageous" to "Compassionate" to "Confident." But I have never heard anyone answer that they want to be "afraid" or "confused."

Who do you want to be?

Personally, I want to be someone who is brave and compassionately committed.

Whatever view you adopt for yourself, whoever you want to be, hold that image in your mind. See and feel yourself as that person. Then dive into the next chapter, mind open, expecting nothing but the best from yourself.

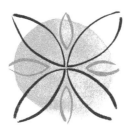

....

Chapter 2

....

Exercise is an Easy Move

The very first thing I did when I was diagnosed with MS was start working out. I still think this is one of the best decisions I've ever made. I gravitated toward working out because it was the quickest action I could take. I wanted to do something immediately to help myself. And I got no discouragement from my doctor when I floated the idea by him. Before then, I'd worked out a smidge—some sports growing up, going for a run now and then, the standard gym membership I used maybe ten times in a year. But none of it was true, habitual, can't-wait-to-do-it working out.

Within a week of my diagnosis, my sister and I joined a gym. Choosing a gym I loved was important to me. Not all gyms are created equal, not to me at least. I knew I was choosing a second home, a place to bond and create new relationships. I found one that fit my personality. It's small, family-owned, has lots of trainers, and everybody knew my name and story. I'm a boutique kind of girl, and I like the feel of small and homey over a giant and impersonal big-box gym where I would stay anonymous.

My sister and I decided to hire a personal trainer as well. We wanted someone to show us what to do, so we could hit the ground running (literally)—no wasting time messing around pretending to know what to do on each machine. Choosing the type of environment I thrived in, and clarifying where my procrastination tended to happen so I could address it directly, were important steps. I had an agenda and I was determined.

And petrified.

When I arrived at the gym on my first day of working out, I sat in my car, engine off, and gave myself a pep talk. I mentally separated myself from thoughts about what I looked like, if I fit in, if my natural clumsiness was going to show up and seriously injure me or my ego. Then I made myself get out of the car and walk into the gym. I know my eyes were huge. I was timid and quiet and I tried to make myself as small as possible.

It's important to note here that as a kid I consistently received the "Talks Too Much to Her Neighbor" award from my teachers. I'm not sure if anyone who's met me would describe me as "timid." In other words, I was acting nothing like myself.

I remember asking the guy at the front desk, "Is Kurt here?" It sounded like I wasn't sure if Kurt was working there that day (which was ridiculous because I knew he was).

Kurt was pointed out, across the room with my sister. It was such a relief to see someone familiar in this completely unfamiliar environment. I let out a breath I hadn't realized I was holding.

Walking across the room to them, my eyes still wide, I tried to take in the busy space where everyone seemed to know exactly what they were doing. Bombarded with new stimuli—the slightly musky smell, the clanks of the equipment, grunts and laughter from all the people who obviously felt at home there—I took my place next to my sister.

Knowing my sister was with me felt just like seeing a friend in a busy cafeteria at lunchtime. My fake-it-'til-you-make-it confidence could relax a bit in the friendly territory, as long as I was with her.

I love that feeling of navigating something so new you can't even process all the pieces, while knowing it will soon feel like second nature. That's what kept me moving forward at the gym. Even though I was terrified of what this new chapter of my life would look like, I knew I would soon be one of the people who looked at home there.

What's Good for Humans

Whenever I teach a workshop for people living with MS, I ask the participants to raise their hands if their doctor has said exercise was bad for them. No hands are ever raised. I would put money on the notion that your doctor has never told you exercise is bad. That's because the benefits of exercise are almost endless. I'm not telling you anything you don't already know.

Exercise affects your mood by acting as a powerful anti-depressant, releasing endorphins, and boosting your spirit. It not only strengthens your muscles, but reduces and possibly reverses the risk of other diseases like obesity and diabetes (unfortunately, having MS doesn't preclude other conditions). Exercise stimulates neurogenesis, which is the production of new neurons in the hippocampus, effectively increasing our capacity for learning and memory. I could go on about the benefits. But, even though we are well aware of the reasons to be (and stay) active, I still often get asked, "Is it ok to work out since I have MS?"

It's a valid question. Even though there are all these studies about the greatness of exercise, they fall short of saying, "Exercise will specifically help *your* MS." That's due to a few factors. First, we live in a society where sneezing in the wrong direction can get you sued. For that reason, very few people have the bravery it takes to say, "This is absolutely proven to help *your* MS. Period. End of story." Second, even if they have that bravery, it's hard to scientifically prove that a specific action will consistently cause a specific result in different people. And, at the next level, that the specific action will give *you* the specific result. That's because MS is such a personal matter. What works for one person may not work at all for someone else.

There are so many factors that go into what your MS looks like: what type of MS you have, your age, what treatment protocol you're on and when you started it (if you started it), fitness, food, stress, etc. It's hard for anyone who's not you to say definitively what will work for you.

Later in this chapter I'll tell you about a vital thing to keep in mind while you're exercising, but for now, here's how I answer the question "Is it ok to work out since I have MS?": Yes. It's ok to exercise with MS. In fact, I believe it's essential. I invite you to ask your doctor right now if you should (especially if you have another diagnosis). Chances are, he or she will say yes. Even if it's difficult to find someone who will say yes without immediately unsaying it, exercise can make *your* MS better.

My belief is that if it's good for humans, it's good for humans with MS.

A Note on Heat

This book is not about telling you what will happen with your MS or any other diagnosis you have. However, I do want to mention something that may come up when you work out. If you're not aware of the possibility, it can be alarming and cause you to think you have to stop. I'm mentioning it because the next question I'm often asked about exercising is, "Will my MS get worse when I'm hot?" There's a reaction to heat that some people with MS get called Uhthoff's Phenomenon. The severity of Uhthoff's varies and some people don't get this reaction at all. Those who do can notice an uptick in their symptoms when they get hot. These are symptoms they've already had that seem to worsen when they're hot. This is not a relapse or your MS getting worse. This is something that happens when your body heats up, like when you work out or have a fever or live in Texas in the summer. Uhthoff's symptoms will fade when you cool down.

Some people take the Uhthoff's Phenomenon to mean they can't work out if they have MS. But there are workarounds so you can still get the benefits of exercise. If you have a problem with heat, focus on staying cool when you work out. For example, exercise early in the day if you're exercising outside, or use cooling towels to help reduce the effects of the heat.

If you think Uhthoff's Phenomenon is happening while you work out, be aware of it. What does it feel like when you get hot? (It may manifest as blurry vision.) If you slow down, do the symptoms go away? Is it better when you do low-impact versus high-impact exercise?

Play around and see what heating up while working out does for you, if anything. Take your reaction to heat as a way to get to know yourself better, not as something to be afraid of. How do you react? Do you react at all?

I still get people I've met for five minutes telling me what my MS will do to me. But I can say that 100 percent of those predictions have been wrong. One of those predictions was that heat would take me out, that it would crush me and leave me on the sidelines for a week. Not true. And it may not be true for you, either. I stay away from extreme heat like hot yoga and being in 100-degree weather for a long time, but that's as far as it goes.

By getting to know what actually does happen to you when you get hot, you won't have to shy away from exercise. And there's a good chance you may reach fitness goals you never thought you could.

Find out Why

There I was. I had my great gym, my trainer to tell me how to get the best results, and my sister there for motivation, love, and support. But having all of that in place wasn't going to make me show up. I was very truthful with myself about that. Those circumstances didn't make me do anything—I could still blow it off if I wanted to.

So why didn't I?

I was clear with myself from the beginning that my sister and my trainer were not "accountability partners." It was my responsibility alone to show up. This was all on me. I showed up for every session, but I didn't depend on someone else holding me accountable. I didn't set up a reward system to entice me to do what I didn't want to do. I didn't even create a mantra to be repeated on days I'd rather stay home and watch trashy TV. I did what Simon Sinek teaches top business people and leaders to do: I started with understanding the very personal reason why I was doing it.

Most of us start with the *what* or the *how*. If you're like me, when you were diagnosed your first question was, "What can I do?" In his book, *Start With Why*, Sinek teaches that what keeps us motivated is not what we do, or even how we do it. It's understanding *why* we do it in the first place.

When you understand your deepest desire of why you're doing something, you create a foundation that never leaves you, a renewable source of motivation.

For me, knowing the goodness I delivered to myself each time I worked out was my why. I knew that with every step I took, my mind and body were getting stronger. I knew that I was repairing myself at a molecular level, and helping my future self. That was my why. And it's kept me going for 15 years.

Why do you want to work out? The most important thing, always, is to be honest with yourself. If you don't want to work out, that's ok. If you're only doing it because you feel like you have to, that's ok, too. There are no wrong answers. But if you're thinking about working out, that means you want to, at least on some level. Connect with that. Why do you think working out is important for you?

We do things because we think we'll benefit from them somehow. How will you benefit from exercising? This may not be a two-second answer for you. When I'm working with clients who are having trouble with this question, I invite them to noodle on it for awhile. Keep asking *why* until you hit on something that gives you a tug. Find that little tug, and then build on it.

Now I have many reasons why I work out, but I started with one: I believed exercising was the best thing I could do for my MS. I still believe that.

Today, I love working out. I run, walk, lift weights, cycle. I've even trained in Jiu Jitsu. I play around with exercising, change it up, and keep it interesting, because I know my personality, and that's what I need in order to thrive. Sometimes I listen to a fun running app and get chased by zombies, and sometimes I stay unplugged and listen to the birds waking up in the morning. I need variety. But no matter what I'm doing, or how I'm doing it, I always focus on why.

It Starts with a Whisper

The second most frequent question I get around exercise is, "What should I do?" First and foremost, do what you love. If you like walking, great. If you're a runner, keep going. If you're new to the whole workout idea to begin with, there are a million things to try—pick one and see how it goes. The most important part of your workout is not what you do (there are great trainers out there to help you with that), it's listening to your body while you're doing it.

Our bodies are constantly talking to us. I love how one of my teachers, Martha Beck, says that our bodies are like animals. They can't verbally tell us what's going on, but they communicate through numerous signs. We can feel the pain of a joint or muscle. We can feel weightless when we're excited.

Once, when I had a severe muscle strain, I could see a physical dent in my quad (yikes is right!). Our bodies talk to us, and we don't have to wait until we see the damage to know what they say. We can learn how to listen to their subtle communications.

Our bodies will always whisper before they yell.

Try It—Body Meditation

A favorite technique I use to listen to my body is a meditation I adapted from Martha Beck. This is something I teach in my program. In this book I'll teach you how to adapt it to pay attention to yourself in many areas. You'll see this technique again, in Chapter 4 and Chapter 7, when I talk about emotions and energy.

To begin, turn off any distractions and get comfortable. You can do this meditation sitting or lying down. Start by closing your eyes and breathing: three deep breaths—in through your nose and out through your mouth.

Pay attention to the top of your head. Notice how it feels. Does it hurt? Does it feel normal? Can you feel it at all? Whatever it is, just notice. Then move down to your forehead. How does it feel? Is it tensed? Relaxed? Again, just notice and move on to your temples. Then notice your cheeks, your jaw, throat, neck, shoulders, arms, back, etc. Slowly move down through your entire body, including your solar plexus, gut, and stomach. Right down to your fingers and toes. As you move through, keep pausing, asking yourself how it feels, and listening to the answer. Just notice everything.

This is not meant to take very long. You can do it in five minutes, or you can take longer. It's up to you. The important thing is that you notice how each part of your body feels. Give yourself time to notice the subtle answers.

You may discover that a part of your body has a dull pain that you hadn't been aware of. You may find that something that has bothered you before is now fine. Start building your foundation of awareness about your body.

I suggest doing this body meditation daily for about a week in order to get a good baseline reading as well as a sense of how to do this in a way that works best for you.

Start right now—take a moment away from reading and try it out for yourself...

You've just started the dialogue between your awareness and your body. Once you've tried this meditation a few times, you can use it when you're working out. This is the *how* in exercise that's so important for keeping your body healthy.

Basic Body Meditation

....

Start a log of body meditations for one week. What stands out on a daily basis? What are the common factors you notice?

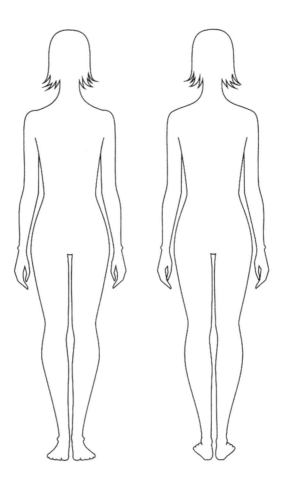

Note areas on the picture and write specifically how each one feels. On a scale of 1–10, how strong is this feeling?

NEED MORE ROOM?

Go to *www.AndreaHansonCoaching.com/BookSheets*
and download your own free Basic Body Meditation and
Workout Body Meditation worksheets.

Honoring What We Hear

When we work out, we're literally applying stress to our bodies. There are different forms of stress, and not all of them are bad. With exercise, we want to push ourselves, we want to do our best, and that means leaving our comfort zones. But how do we know the difference between a "good" push that leaves us energized and a "bad" push that will leave us energized and a "bad" push that will leave a dent in our quad? The answer lies in listening first, and then in honoring what we hear.

I was working with a client who loves cycling. She had done the body meditation earlier in the week during a bike ride, and noticed about halfway through the ride that her body was tensing up. Her hands and legs had a specific feel to them. I asked her, "What was your body telling you in that moment?" She thought for a second, remembered that overall feeling in her body, and said, "You know, it was telling me to keep going. I knew that at that point in the ride I was close to a hump and I just need to get over it, so I knew I would feel fine soon."

That's the type of awareness you get when you're fully paying attention to what your body says.

As you work out, take an inventory of how your body feels. After the first ten minutes, run through a body meditation. When you've practiced it a few times and gotten the hang of it, you'll find you can do this pretty easily while still moving (and without anyone noticing). Do the body meditation again, halfway through your workout, and also at the end. In this way, not only will you notice how your body is feeling while you work out, you'll also really start to know how your body feels while you're physically pushing yourself.

Use the body meditation every time you work out. As you do the body meditation, ask yourself "Is my body saying to stop or to keep going?" Sometimes your body will say, "Go! This is awesome!" and sometimes it will say, "Slow it down."

Pay attention not only to the parts of your body, but the overall feeling in your body. For me, when I'm in push-it mode, my body feels light and bouncy. The workout is tough, but there's airiness in how I move. But my body can switch into slow-it-down mode on a dime. Then I feel heavier on my feet and I feel my form start to break down slightly. That's my cue to slow down or stop.

What are your cues? How does your body tell you to keep on pushing? How does it tell you to slow it down? At first, you may only notice a cue when it's pretty obvious. You probably already have a good idea if you think about how your body feels when you have to stop. That's a great starting point. But try to notice it a little sooner each time. This is how you find your body's whispers before they get loud (and turn into something painful).

Once you get used to hearing your body communicate, ask yourself the question: "Am I honoring what my body's telling me?"

When I badly strained my quad, I heard my body telling me to slow down long before the strain happened. But I didn't honor it. I didn't slow down. Sometimes we don't slow down when we know we should. The interesting part is observing why we don't.

For me, back then, I had something to prove to myself. I was insecure with where I was physically. I thought if I could get to a certain level in my running, I would be worthy. Worthy of being a runner. Worthy of being healthy. If I got to that level of worthiness, it would mean that the MS wasn't beating me. That's the irony in why we don't listen. We think we're losing if we listen, but actually we lose big when we don't.

Our bodies will always tell us what we need to know. We can learn to listen and choose whether we want to honor the message. When we hear the whisper, we can do something easy and immediate to fix the issue. When our body gets louder, we can be benched while we heal. But when our body screams, that's when bad things can happen, especially with MS.

My personal goal is to never let my body get to that screaming point again. The good news is it doesn't ever have to.

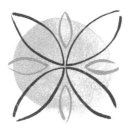

Chapter 3

The Art of Eavesdropping

S tacey, a client of mine, and I had a very intense discussion. She wanted me to agree that her future job was going to be hard. She laid out all her very logical reasons. She had a few examples from her past that proved it had been hard before. So, naturally, it would be hard again. She begged me to agree to this *one simple point*, to validate that her new job would, in fact—no two ways about it—be hard. She made a very well-presented case. But I didn't buy it.

"No, I won't agree with that." I told her.

"Come *on*, anyone would agree that it would be hard."

"Not true. I don't."

"Just a little bit hard? You'll admit that, right?"

"I will not."

"Seriously?"

"Nope."

This discussion went on in a similar way until we were laughing about it. Stacey laughed because she started to realize the absurdity of wanting so badly to hear this one bit of validation from me. I laughed, not only because she was wickedly funny in her presentation, but also because I knew nothing she said would make me agree that her new job would be hard. Especially because, at that point, her new job was only theoretical.

Everyone looks at things a little bit differently and has his or her own definitions and framework for decision-making. In our conversation, Stacey and I had different views of what "hard" means, and different views about whether something being hard is good or bad. We were both right. The way we viewed her theoretical job was personal to each of us. We choose whether to see things as hard or easy. We choose whether to think something "hard" could be exhilarating, or would slowly cause a breakdown.

There's no rule.

That's what my client discovered as we talked. By believing the new job would be hard and stress her out, she was creating her reality. Whatever that job would entail, her thoughts would make it seem hard, and that's why she was going to be stressed. She couldn't understand why that wasn't my reality, because she had convinced herself so deeply that her thoughts were facts of life. They weren't facts to me at all. I chose to see things differently. Stacey was learning that she could make that choice, too.

There's a good reason Stacey believed so strongly in what she thought. She had believed for a long time that *jobs are hard*. We all have such beliefs—ideas we take as fact and never question, because we don't think there is any question. Perhaps past experiences have taught us those beliefs, and we continue to apply them to everything. Maybe we think everyone feels the same way because we hear those messages from others, too.

There have been quite a few things I've believed were facts and didn't question. Like my client, I once thought those things were the truth. I'll give you some examples. I believed my boss was stressing me out. If I went to another company, my life would be better. If I lost the weight, ate the right food, got fit, everything in my life will be easier. I would feel so much relief if I had more money. I even (albeit briefly) had moments where I knew life would be more enjoyable if I had a man.

Because I believed so deeply that those statements were fact, I was constantly disappointed. If you'd asked me how I felt then, I would have said I felt trapped—because the diets didn't work or the weight didn't come off quickly enough. I was exhausted because other people were *always* starting drama. I was stressed out because of my job. And I was so afraid that I would run out of money or that my MS would take a wrong turn.

I took action and did what I thought I had to do to feel better. Only it never worked out as planned. I got a different job and things were great, until new stressors popped up. I lost a ton of weight and felt great, until I realized my life wasn't really that different. I dated quite a few guys. It was fun, until I realized that none were marriage material. I followed the advice of many nutritionists who told me what would work to help me lose weight and help me with my MS. Their advice was often contradictory. I cycled through all sorts of food restrictions: gluten-free, dairy-free, sugar-free, yeast-free. I was always more miserable than before.

In fact, I felt worse when I tried to force the changes I thought would improve my life. I remember crying at night, frustrated about making myself keep to the latest strict diet, thinking I had no choice if I wanted to be happy.

I felt absolutely powerless, because I *knew* that if those things changed, I would feel better. But I also knew I had little control over changing them. I was stuck in a cycle of scanning my life for potential changes so I could feel healthier and better, but then not feeling any different after making huge changes. And I did all of that while telling myself I was completely Zen and believing it was up to me to be happy. It was all very contradictory and excessive. And I was miserable.

Change of Regime

I first started working with my mentor, Brooke Castillo, in 2011. I love the irony that, in searching for the life changes that would make me feel better, I chose a mentor who taught me that my that life didn't have to be any different than it already was in order to change how I felt about it. Although I believe this 100 percent now, it took time to process this way of thinking.

Brooke taught me the difference between knowing something intellectually and truly owning it. Intellectually, I knew that only I could make myself happy. Intellectually, I knew that I needed to keep a positive attitude. But I still expected other people and other things in my life to change in order for me to experience that happiness and that positive attitude.

When I started learning from Brooke, I protested and threw tantrums and defended the fact (or so I thought it was a fact) that I felt exhausted because of my career choice or my weight or anything else going on. I will admit that I still protest and have tantrums, and I encourage my clients to do the same. Changing your mindset can be like a change of regime, and a healthy internal debate is an important part of the switchover. Sometimes we must simply thrash around before we can accept something new, even if the new thing is a change that we want.

I was convinced that my job was stressing me out. I worked in finance, and there was plenty of evidence that my career path would give me ulcers. I believed the thought that I had to get out of that job *first*, and *then* I could focus on me. But Brooke wouldn't agree. In fact she wouldn't even let me list all the evidence I had of why my life was crazy. "All that evidence doesn't matter," she told me.

Like Stacey when she was trying to convince me that her job would be hard, I started to understand what Brooke was showing me.

Viewing my job as crazy and stressful and draining was only one way I could choose to see my situation. As I broke my thoughts down, I realized there were many different ways I could perceive my job. For example, my job was eye-opening, challenging, and life-changing. And even if it was stressful, that stress didn't have to be a bad thing. My mind was blown when I had all these new thoughts about my job. I saw that even though they were different, and painted a very different picture, they were also true.

Let's Break This Down

On a basic level, a thought is simply a perspective about something. For example, I think the color yellow is pretty. Someone else may think yellow is ok, but blue is beautiful. These are only thoughts expressed as sentences that describe opinions.

Thoughts aren't who we are. I am not defined by the fact that I think yellow is pretty. If I *were* my thought, I would have an identity crisis every time I changed my mind. Which pretty much means I would be in crisis daily. Thankfully, that's not how it works.

Thoughts can change. We change our minds all the time. I can think that yellow isn't so pretty anymore. What I choose to think is entirely my choice. Yellow doesn't *make* me think it's pretty. I don't have to like it if I see it. I have the choice, always, to think what I want to think.

Our minds are constantly commenting on the world around us, offering opinions about this and that, like whether we think something is funny or beautiful or irrelevant. These are all only thoughts. Our brains have tens of thousands of thoughts running through them each day, some we share out loud, some we keep to ourselves, some are so familiar we may not realize we thought them at all until we actively observe them. Our thoughts are not all unique thoughts. A lot of them are repeated over and over again in our heads. This is why we feel like some thoughts are so true they don't warrant questioning. The human brain wants to be correct in what it's thinking and when our brains are consistently presented with the same thought, we believe that it's correct. When we have strong beliefs, strong physical connections are formed in our brains around those neural pathways. This is why it can be so hard to convince someone that what he or she thinks is a fact is actually not true at all.

Take, for example, the thought that creating new habits is hard. When I believe that thought, it forms a groove my brain. Each time I think about new habits being hard to create, that groove gets deeper until it's something I don't even question. I think it all the time, with conviction. Eventually, a channel forms that this belief can flow through very quickly and easily. Our brains are nothing if not efficient. Using this well-dug channel is the most efficient path there is. Therefore, there's no reason to question the belief that flows through it. I think it very easily. *New habits? Hard to create.* I don't have to think very long or very hard about it. I just *know* it. Which is to say, I believe it.

Forcing yourself to believe something different takes effort, because it involves working against our own neural channels. To believe, instead, that new habits are easy to create, I would need to develop a whole different groove. When I do, that groove is not as deep at first. The once-efficient flow of thought on this topic of habits becomes a small trickle, and my mind won't go there readily, because our minds like efficiency. And this small trickle of a new thought isn't efficient—at first.

Although our thoughts aren't who we are, they're very important. Understanding what we believe about something is essential, because what we think shapes how we feel and, in turn, that affects how we react.

Think about the color yellow again. If you're in a room with yellow walls and your thought about yellow is you like it, you may feel comfortable in that room, even happy. You will stay in that room without protest. But if you're in that same room and your thought about yellow is that it's heinous, you will feel uncomfortable and leave as soon as you can. The color didn't *make* you take action and leave. The walls didn't push you out. What you thought about the wall color determined how you felt in that room and how you reacted to it.

One little thought can determine so much. To find out what we think about something isn't hard. We don't have to dig into our subconscious. We only have to pay closer attention by eavesdropping on our thoughts.

Try It—Thought Storm Exercise

Your thoughts may feel like they're storming in your head, especially if you have lots of opinions or are in a conflict. The thoughts you have can feel very forceful and real. This exercise, adapted from one of the very first exercises I did with my mentor Brooke Castillo, is a way to begin becoming more aware of what you think.

Think of something or someone in your life. It can be your job, your spouse, your kids, or something else. When learning to observe thoughts, it may be easier to work with something seemingly insignificant, like the shirt you're wearing, or the chair you're sitting on. Take out a fresh piece of paper and write for three minutes on what you think about that topic. Write down anything that comes to mind. Don't judge what you write, or even edit it for grammar. Just get it down. This is a thought storm.

Here's an example. If I were writing about traffic, my thought storm would look like this: *It's loud. I hate it. It's a pain. It costs me money in gas. It's unnecessary. All of these people should be at work instead of on the road.*

People don't know how to drive. The reason there's traffic is because of all this construction, which should have been taken care of by now.

Each sentence here is a thought.

Your turn. Write down what you think about your topic and get a nice list of thoughts.

Next, beside each thought, write down whether it's fact or opinion. Facts are objective. For example, *Sitting in traffic costs money in gas.* That's a fact. But *People don't know how to drive*, although it seems like a fact, is an opinion. It's not true for all people, and *don't know how to drive* is a subjective judgment. I may have a much lower threshold than someone else of what I consider to be "bad" driving. This is an opinion.

Thought Storm

....

Pick a topic (it can be anything) and write about it for three minutes straight. Do not edit, judge or change grammatical errors.

Topic: _____

Thoughts about topic:

_____

_____

_____

_____

_____

_____

_____

_____

_____

_____

Read over what you wrote. Underline each sentence that's an opinion. What do you notice?

_____

_____

_____

_____

_____

_____

_____

GET YOUR OWN THOUGHT STORM WORKSHEET!
Go to *www.AndreaHansonCoaching.com/BookSheets*
and download your free worksheet.

Go through your list and highlight all the opinions. These are actually thoughts. They determine how you feel and react to the something or someone you're thinking about. What do you notice about your thoughts now that you're looking at them? Are there any surprises?

For me, this exercise showed that I had been aware on a basic level of what I thought about traffic: didn't like it, waste of my time. The more I looked at what I'd written down about it, the more I realized the sheer number of thoughts I had—and just how bitter I was—about traffic. In turn, each of those thoughts made me feel something and spurred a reaction in me.

As I began practicing being aware of my thoughts in general, a few things happened. First, I was appalled at some of them. I couldn't believe how many of my thoughts were negative and just plain mean (often towards myself). Second, I realized that no matter how overwhelmed I was by them, they weren't new thoughts at all. I wasn't all of a sudden creating them. I was only switching off the autopilot so that I could pay attention to what was really going on in my noggin.

It turned out there were a lot of thoughts I hadn't even realized I was having. It became crystal clear that the thoughts in my head were shaping not only how I viewed the world, but also how I felt about and reacted to events.

If my thoughts determine so much, and if I can change them when I want to, that means my topic—my circumstance, the things I'm thinking about—has nothing to do with how I feel and how I react. I can change my mind a hundred times, but the topic I'm thinking about doesn't have to change even slightly for me to begin to feel differently about it and react differently to it.

What Does This Have to Do with My MS?

My single biggest breakthrough came when I realized that my MS was only a circumstance, and only one part of my world that I have opinions about. My MS doesn't *make* me feel fear or shame or guilt. My MS doesn't *make* me worry about the what-ifs that might happen down the road. I *choose* to think about them. My MS doesn't *make* me feel defeated when I have a flare-up. I feel defeated when I think having a flare-up means I'll never get better. Nor does my MS make me feel happy when everything is going well. I feel happy when I believe I'm in control. My MS doesn't make me feel flaky when I back out of plans. I feel that when I think I'm being a bad friend.

When I hear a prediction that MS will do something bad to me, it's not my MS making me feel upset. It's not even the person telling me the story who makes me feel upset. It's me, if I choose to believe what they're saying.

My thoughts, not my MS, are the hub of all of my feelings. I choose the thoughts I keep.

And that's a beautiful thing.

What about You?

Have you started practicing how to become aware of your thoughts? If so, what have you learned about how much clout your thoughts have, how they drive the way you feel and react to your world? In Chapter 1, I wrote about how important expectations are. Guess what? Expectations are thoughts, too. Very important ones.

What do you think about your MS? What do you expect from it?

I encourage you to take some time to think about your answer to that question, or even to do a thought storm about your MS, because all the answers that come up for you will be useful. All of your answers are what you expect to happen with your MS, whether you say them out loud to yourself or not.

When we first start working together, I often ask clients what they think of their MS. I get two distinct types of answers: what they say out loud, and what they believe in their gut. What they say out loud to other people about their MS is often something like, "It's a challenge, but I'll get through it." But then there are the answers they don't speak out loud. Or maybe they only say when they're confiding in someone they really trust. Maybe they don't even admit them to themselves, because they've judged them as wrong or bad or too scary or not positive.

The answers you don't speak out loud are important ones, because those are what you most believe. They're thoughts you're acting on, even if you didn't know about them until you took a closer look.

Keep asking yourself the question, *What do I think about my MS?* Keep examining your answer. The answer you believe deep in your gut may surprise you. And it may help you.

MS is very personal, so our thoughts about it are going to be very personal. Looking at both types of answers you give to the question—what you tell others and what you don't say out loud—can be eye-opening. The thoughts you tell other people may not always be positive and the thoughts in your gut may not always be negative, so try not to make assumptions about what you'll find as you become more aware of your thoughts.

For a long time, I gave the "It sucks, but I'll beat it" answer when people asked me about my MS. I especially felt like I had to give that answer to other people with MS. But hidden beneath that façade and a generous layer of self-doubt was the knowledge in my gut that everything would be ok. I was afraid of that answer and squashed it for many years. I assumed it was an arrogant thought and would jinx me if I spoke it out loud. Or maybe it would cause too much conflict with someone else.

Eventually, I accepted what having MS means to me. Now, I love it that I've always deeply known I will be ok. My hope is that this is what your gut tells you as well. Don't miss out on the opportunity to find out what your gut tells you by following your thoughts to greater awareness. Then use that greater awareness of what you think, and your power to choose different thoughts as needed, to make your life even better.

....

Chapter 4

....

How To Do Emotions

"I can't start that now. What if I have a bad reaction?" my client, Renée, asked during our discussion about a new medication her neurologist recommended.

"Answer your own question." I suggested. "What if you do have a bad reaction?"

"Then I may have to stay home for a while until I feel better."

"And what if you do have to stay home? What happens then?" I pushed her a bit further.

"My boss hates it when I'm out. He may fire me!"

"What if he does?" I kept going with Renée's predictions of what would happen in this purely theoretical situation.

"Then I'll have no paycheck. I won't be able to pay my bills." Her speech quickened and got a bit defensive, as if to say, "How can you ask such questions? Clearly all this will happen."

"What if you don't pay your bills? Then what?" I continued.

"I'll lose my house. I'll have no income."

"Then what do you think you'll do? What will happen?"

"I'll be homeless and it will be awful." She said this with disbelief that I didn't know the answer already.

I have conversations like this with clients all the time. The conversation starts with a fear of doing something new that takes a bit of courage. Within five minutes, their scenario of what will happen when things go wrong escalates to an ending that usually includes being homeless or put out financially. Life coach and author Martha Beck says our greatest fears always boil down to becoming a bag lady. I agree. Exposing that fear of becoming a bag lady is why I keep asking clients what they think will happen when they're afraid of something new. I do it so they can witness how easily they assume they'll be helpless and poor if they take a risk.

After Renée told me she would become homeless, she was quiet for a moment, reflecting on what she had just said. Then I summarized the chain of events to her. "So," I said calmly, "What you're saying is if you try this new drug, you will become bankrupt and friendless. Is that what you believe?"

Renée let out a breath. She saw the downward spiral. Most importantly, she saw that she had assumed her inevitable helplessness in this situation. Renée is a go-getter, very smart and resourceful. This rolling over and playing dead is not part of her personality at all.

"Actually, it's *not* true." she said with more conviction. "I would handle it. I would get another job. I would ask people for help. I would figure something out."

"So, what about the new meds?" I asked.

"They may be totally fine. My doctor told me that this medication is well-tolerated. If I do have a reaction, I'll deal with it."

Then she started laughing, "Wow—I can't believe I thought I would be homeless!"

Fear: Billions of People Served

Why is this story of assuming bankruptcy and being alone so common? It's because when we decide that something bad will result from something unknown, we become afraid. And feeling afraid leads to acting afraid.

Renée did what we all tend to do when we're focusing on feeling afraid. She forgot a few crucial pieces of the story. First, she forgot that her doctor said the medication was well-tolerated. Second, she forgot that her very nature is to get back up and fight when things go wrong.

When Renée allowed her fear to take control, she couldn't see how things could be better. I love conversations like the one I had with her because often, when acting out of fear, we don't even question the fear we began with. When Renée kept talking about what she thought would happen, she eventually realized she'd described a pretty irrational chain of events, one that left out key pieces of information. But if she hadn't verbalized what she thought and ultimately seen the truth, she would have gone on and lived with those beliefs instead of questioning them. She would have stayed afraid of her new meds and probably not tried them. Or she would have taken the medication, but with the expectation of something bad happening. None of those scenarios would have resulted in Renée feeling in control.

Renée decided to look at her new medication differently. She knew there was a low chance of her having a bad reaction. And if she did, she knew she would deal with it. She was actually feeling excited to take the new medication and believed it held a lot of promise for her.

She tolerated the medication beautifully and is still on it today. This outcome was possible because she gained control of her inner situation.

Renée's story shows how powerful our emotions are. The decision she faced about taking a new medication didn't change. How she *felt* about the decision did change. In actuality, *what* she was afraid of didn't matter at all. She could have been afraid of a tiger instead of a new medication and had a similar reaction. Fear was the factor that drove her actions.

What is fear? What is powerlessness? They feel very real, palpable, and even tangible. But fear is only an emotion, not a fact. Powerlessness is an emotion. Excitement is an emotion. So are joy and peacefulness. Emotions drive our reactions.

Our motivation for nearly all we do boils down to wanting to stop feeling bad or to feel better. Test this out for yourself: Why are you reading this book? Your answer may be because this book can help you manage your MS. Why do you want to manage your MS? Probably because you want to stay healthy. Why do you want to stay healthy? If you're like me, your answer is because it's better to be healthy and in control of your MS management than to do nothing. But why is being in control better? Because *it feels better* to have that control instead of doing nothing. Ultimately, feeling better and feeling in control are likely driving your decision to read this book.

One Small Problem

Generally, we want to feel good. We've heard all the fuss about the importance of positive attitudes, and we want to be happy. We don't like to be afraid, upset, or helpless, and so we do what we can to avoid feeling that way. But there's one small problem with that. In the process of trying to feel better, we tend to give control of how we feel over to other people and circumstances. We saw an example of that in how

Renée initially thought that using the new medication would cause her to feel helpless and afraid.

We can mistakenly give away control of our emotions like a gift, wrapped in a bow. Often when we're dealing with something big, like having MS, it's as if we're saying, "Here, MS. You take control. Let me know how I'll feel today. I know I have no choice here."

If the reason we do things is because we want to feel better, or at least not feel worse, what happens when we don't think we have any power over how we feel? Ironically, we create the feeling of not being in control when we believe we don't have control over how we feel. That's a pretty awful catch-22.

Renée thought she had no choice but to feel helpless if she took the new meds. If I had asked her at the beginning of our session how she wanted to feel about deciding to take new meds, she would have said something like "calm" or "confident." At that time, she believed that how she felt emotionally wasn't up to her, but was dependent on how her body reacted to the medication.

The beautiful thing is that this lack of control over how you feel isn't real.

If we've given away control, then it's ours to take back. And that's what we must do for our emotional well-being. How we feel emotionally is completely our choice, not only when things are easy and going well, but on our worst of the worst days. Feeling happy doesn't happen automatically because things are going well. Just like feeling petrified doesn't happen automatically because things take a wrong turn. How we feel, always, depends on our perspectives about the situation.

Try It—Flash Cash

Imagine that you're walking down the sidewalk and a well-dressed woman comes up to you and gives you $500 cash. She smiles, tells you the money is for you, and then walks away.

What would you think if that happened to you?

When running this exercise with clients, I get answers of anything from, "I'm blessed!" to, "Who is this person and is this money real?"

Try it. List all the thoughts you would have if the scenario with the $500 happened to you. Try to write at least six different thoughts.

Now look at the thoughts you wrote down. What emotion did each of your thoughts make you feel? For example, if you think you're being duped into accepting fake cash, you'll likely feel annoyed or angry, not peaceful and loving. If you think you're lucky and want to pay this surprise bounty forward, you'll likely feel excited or happy instead of upset. Play around with the different thoughts you observe and try to match up feelings with each one.

Next, take out a fresh piece of paper. Write down the following emotions: suspicious, overjoyed, upset, annoyed, and peaceful. Determine what you would need to *think* about the stranger giving you the $500 cash in order to feel each of those emotions.

For example, to feel annoyed, my thought might be, *This must be a trick. I don't have time for this* or *Where's the camera? I don't want to be on TV with this hair.* Try to think of thoughts that make you feel suspicious, overjoyed, upset, annoyed, and peaceful.

By the end of this exercise, you will have at least 10 different thoughts about a stranger giving you $500, and you can see how each thought can produce a very different emotion.

Review everything you've written down. There are lots of different emotions that come up, and different ways to think about the stranger with the $500. But take a look at what hasn't changed at all. The original premise or circumstance of the stranger coming up to you and giving you $500 has remained the same the whole time. Notice whether you tried to change that original story in your answers about what you thought and felt. Sometimes a client will say that the stranger was wearing ripped clothes, or was acting shifty. But that's not the story. When you do this exercise, keep the original story intact and you will see that the circumstance doesn't need to change in order for you to have different opinions and emotions about it.

Flash Cash

....

Try to think of six thoughts you may have about this scenario. (Ex: "I'm blessed." "Who is this crazy person?" "Is this money real?")

_____

_____

_____

_____

_____

_____

_____

Look at the thoughts you wrote down, and then determine what emotion you feel when you think each thought (ex: Thought: "I'm lucky" Emotion: excited).

Thought: _____

Emotion: _____

Thought: _____

Emotion: _____

Thought: _____

Emotion: _____

Thought: _____

Emotion: _____

Thought: _____

Emotion: _____

Flash Cash (Part Two)

....

Determine what you need to think about the stranger giving you $500 in order to feel each of those emotions.

Emotion: Suspicious
Thought: _____

_____

_____

Emotion: Overjoyed
Thought: _____

_____

_____

Emotion: Upset
Thought: _____

_____

_____

Emotion: Annoyed
Thought: _____

_____

_____

Emotion: Peaceful
Thought: _____

_____

_____

You now have at least ten different thoughts and emotions created about a single situation.

DO YOU WANT A SIMPLE WAY TO DO THE FLASH CASH EXERCISE?

Visit *www.AndreaHansonCoaching.com/BookSheets* to download your own free worksheet with a special bonus section.

Ruby Slipper

The Flash Cash exercise example illustrates a concept that's constant across all situations in life. There are a million opinions to have about a million situations in your world, and each opinion creates an emotion. The circumstance itself doesn't have to change a bit for you to feel differently about it.

Whether you feel good or bad or indifferent is all up to you.

When I realized that how I felt emotionally was 100 percent my choice, I was overjoyed. It's a big responsibility, but we always have the option of what to think about our situation. Once you fully own your emotions, knowing that you're always in control of them is one of the most freeing feelings you can have.

The Positive Mindset

Taking full ownership of how we feel is a very powerful position. So what about when we feel bad? What if we're scared or sad? Should we change our thoughts to happy ones so we can feel happy? I get that question a lot as clients practice emotional awareness. My answer is always, "Not so fast."

A positive mindset is very important. It has been proven that we think faster, more creatively, and we even physically see more things in our environment when we think and feel positively. Having said that, I don't think negative emotions are bad. In fact, I'm tempted to write "positive" and "negative" in quotations because I don't believe there are positive and negative emotions. They're all simply emotions. They're physical sensations we feel in our bodies. When we're happy, we laugh. When we're sad we may feel a lump in our throat. When we're nervous, we can feel a pit in our stomach. Whether emotions are bad or good are labels we place on them to signal the meanings we've attached to them.

When we allow ourselves to feel emotions, those feelings don't actually last very long. Think about the last time you had a good belly laugh. You didn't suppress it, I'm guessing. You let yourself laugh out loud for as long as it was funny. How long was that laugh? A few seconds? A minute? Maybe closer to two minutes? How long was it before you quieted down, the laughter subsided, and you were left with a smile? As Jill Bolte Taylor, author of *My Stroke of Insight*, discovered, 90 seconds is about how long it takes for an emotion to run through the body. All emotions work the same way. If we let ourselves have a good cry, how long does that last before it subsides? About 90 seconds.

Emotions, no matter what they are, need to be felt. They're meant to run through us and then subside. It's ok to have a negative emotion. Relax into it and let the feeling happen.

The reason negative emotions seem to last longer is because we consider it bad to feel them (because if we feel them, we're not being positive). We try to push what we think of as negative emotions away and distract ourselves by staying busy, or we try to deflect negative feelings by forcing ourselves to think of something positive instead.

Remember the channels of habitual thought in our brains, from Chapter 3? It's hard to force ourselves to think of something different—especially if it's the exact opposite of what we believe. When we're feeling sad, it can be tempting to think we should be able to immediately change our mindset and think more positively; then we will feel better. But that can lead to prolonging the sadness because we're resisting it, instead of letting it flow through. We're also forcing positive thoughts we don't truly believe. At that point, we're not actually practicing a positive mindset. We're forcing ourselves to believe something we don't actually believe, trying hard to separate from our bodies and not feel what's really going on, and we're probably doing this while having some thoughts and judgment about having a negative thought in the first place. All this can make us feel anxious and out of sorts.

When we do this, we're white knuckling our way to happiness.

Try It—Emotions Body Meditation

One of the reasons we're so keen to get away from the "negative" feelings is that they don't feel comfortable. Shame is not a snuggly feeling, and neither is guilt or regret. But, just as when you looked at your thoughts and understood them better, once you understand your emotions, they aren't such a scary enigma either. You can come to better understand your emotions by adding a twist to the body meditation that you learned in Chapter 2.

First, what emotion are you feeling right now? It can be anything—happy, calm, scared, whatever. Even if your answer is, "Nothing," I want you to notice how "nothing" feels in your body.

Begin the body meditation by noticing how your head feels, then your throat and shoulders. Notice your solar plexus, your stomach, and your gut. Do you feel heavy or light in those places? Are there parts of your body that feel cold or hot? Check in with your entire body and tune in to what you're feeling physically as you feel emotionally.

One of the times I did this, I noticed that shame feels like ants crawling around my in stomach. It's not a fun feeling, but it wasn't so bad once I understood it. From that point on, shame was no longer a phantom icky feeling anymore, and I could name it. *Oh, I'm feeling shame right now. I feel it in my stomach.* What's interesting is that then I didn't have such a strong need to get away from it anymore (my way of getting away from shame was eating an entire bag of cheesy poofs). I found that once I knew what shame was, and pinpointed the exact feeling of it in my body, I could sit with it until the emotion ran through me. Then I could look at why I was feeling the shame to begin with.

YOU'LL WANT TO DO THIS MORE THAN ONCE.
Visit *www.AndreaHansonCoaching.com/BookSheets* to download the free detailed Emotion Body Meditation worksheet to help you keep track of your progress.

Give Yourself Time

Before Claudia started tuning in to her emotions and how they showed up physically for her, she had been distracting herself and stuffing her feelings down to the point where she honestly had no idea what she was feeling. Even when saying, "I'm really pissed that I have MS," she seemed to feel nothing. I asked her to describe what "nothing" felt like in her body. At first, she couldn't find the feeling in her body. "Nothing feels like nothing," she said. But she stuck with it. She got quiet, did the body meditation, and paid attention.

"There's something in my stomach, like a rock," she said after a few minutes. "It feels hot and heavy." I asked her what emotion that was, and after a minute she said, "Mad, I think. I'm just mad." I asked her to keep feeling it, and she described how mad felt in more detail. "My muscles are tense and my jaw is clenched." After a few minutes of noticing how that felt, she couldn't feel it any longer. The feeling had dissipated because she had simply allowed it and noticed how it felt in her body. Allowing emotion to run through her body led to opening up about her opinions of her MS and her situation.

Eventually, Claudia was able to create a whole new story about her MS, one that helped her feel motivated and in control instead of stuck in an angry feeling that masqueraded as "nothing."

Adding It Up

This chapter has been a crash course in understanding emotions, which is a big topic. Learning that I had control of my own emotions was one of the biggest things I learned from my mentor, Brooke Castillo. Starting your practice of what Brooke calls *emotional maturity* will be a game-changer for you, too.

How do you want to feel about your MS? Do you want to feel powerful? Calm? Peaceful? Do you want to feel motivated? How you feel emotionally about your MS has nothing to do with the MS itself. What you feel doesn't depend on what your MS is doing at the moment. You're in control. You can choose to feel anything you want.

How you want to feel about your MS is an important question to ask yourself because the answer can either set the stage for incredible leaps or stop you in your tracks. The beauty is: You choose.

Keep asking yourself this question: *How do I want to feel about my MS?* Tune in to how you feel and imagine how you want to feel. If the way you feel emotionally is at the core of why you do anything, taking control can change everything.

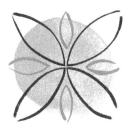

....

Chapter 5

....

Taking the Stress Down a Notch

The first day of the Bike MS event was almost over. Over two days, thousands of people cycled from north Dallas to Fort Worth in a fundraiser for the National MS Society. We rode roughly 80 miles a day. For someone like me, who was not at all a cyclist, it was tough. I could have made the bike ride a little easier on myself by training for more than a few months beforehand, but that's not typically my style. I like to jump into things, and usually that means skipping the recommended preparations.

But I signed up for the event anyway. I biked the whole first day. And then I was exhausted. At my team's tent, I pleaded to a colleague,

"I can't do this again tomorrow!" I was ready to quit. Seriously. "I can't get up tomorrow morning and do what I just did today. It's going to be physically impossible." My legs were like jelly and I didn't even feel like I fully inhabited my body by that point. I felt more like I was floating above it.

My colleague looked me square in the eye, gripped my shoulders, and gave me some of the best advice I've ever received. She said, "Don't think about tomorrow. Just think about what you have to do right now."

Genius.

She was right. When I stood there completely exhausted and thought about the next day, I felt there was no way I would be able to go another 80 miles. That made me want to give up. But the fact was, at that moment, I wasn't doing the second day yet. I was still only doing the end of the first day.

When I imagined what the second day would be like and assumed I would feel then as I did in this moment, I was attached to my prediction that I would fall over and give up. But I was *imagining*. None of my predictions were real yet, because it wasn't tomorrow. When I focused on what I needed right then, *that* was doable. I needed dinner. I needed to sleep for a good eight hours. Those things were easy. I could do them. There was nothing stressful about them.

Something amazing happened when I got some food and a good sleep. By the next morning, I was ready to get on my bike again. At the starting line, I focused on the first ten miles and getting to the rest stop. Then I focused on the next ten miles, and then the next ten miles. I did that all the way to the finish line.

What my colleague had done was pull me back into the present, back from imagining all the grief to come in the future, back to what was actually happening in that very moment.

What happens in the present is the only reality we have.

No matter how much evidence we muster, we don't know what the future holds. Even if we think we have an educated guess, the future surprises us. In contrast, what's happening right here and now is real. When we stay present and focused on what's happening now, things are doable, and we find that we're actually ok. When we try to predict what will happen in the future—like I tried to predict how I would do on the next day of the bike ride—we start to get nervous and afraid. We predict we will fail. We stress out.

By focusing on the current moment, I kept my counterproductive thoughts to a minimum, which is helpful when our thoughts make us want to hide.

I'm eating dinner. Fact.

I'm going to bed. Fact.

I won't be able to get on my bike in the morning and will fail miserably, possibly while people are pointing and laughing at me. Thought.

When I focused on the present, I focused on the facts of the situation. As we saw in Chapter 3, the facts of a situation are objective. No question about it. When you think about how the facts feel, it's often a pretty neutral feeling. Facts are facts and they don't spur any huge emotions.

Thoughts, on the other hand, are subjective. When we think thoughts, they definitely spur emotions. When I thought I would quit the next day, I felt horrible, because I thought I was going to do something I didn't really want to do: walk away from a challenge.

Stress Patrol

All stress is not created equal. Although there are different schools of thought on the different types of stress, I like to break stress down into the two simple categories: voluntary and involuntary.

Involuntary stress arises from factors we don't really have control over, like stress on our bodies from aging or from having a disease like

MS. (There is still no consensus on what causes MS, but scientists do know it's caused by interplay between our genes and our environment. Once we're diagnosed with MS, what we did or didn't do to get it no longer matters. Therefore, I choose to call MS an involuntary stress.) Another type of involuntary stress comes when our bodies are going through a healing process from an injury or sickness.

Voluntary stress is what I want to focus on here, because the majority of stress in everyday life is voluntary. Some voluntary stresses are good, like when we work out, creating physical stress in our bodies to make them stronger. We can also use stress in small doses as motivation. An acute *I'd better get this done* stress, like when finishing a project, can be helpful. Some people thrive on that type of stress, but a shot of that type of stress doesn't last long—it's over as soon as we find the motivation we need.

Some aspects of voluntary stress stick with us and don't help us at all—like when I worry about a deadline for weeks on end, or when I'm afraid of what the next day of bike riding will bring. These are voluntary ideas I'm stressing out about and it's my choice to worry.

In Chapter 3, I brought up the idea that my MS doesn't control my fear. MS doesn't *make* me afraid. My thoughts about MS do. I don't know about you, but being afraid of MS stresses me out. And that's entirely voluntary.

When I work with clients in my program, managing stress is something we always pay attention to. That's because 1) everyone has stress and 2) stress is the top thing doctors tell us to stop doing when we're diagnosed. I've always loved that irony: Here's a crazy disease I have, and I don't know what will happen because of it, but don't stress out about it because that will only make it worse! Ugh.

The good news is that there *is* something you can do about stress. And that's double good, because stressing less is good for dealing with MS and good for humans in general.

Three Types of Voluntary Stress

I break voluntary stress down into three categories: trying to predict the future, being in other people's business, and arguing with reality.

Trying to predict the future. This is what I did at the end of the first day of biking for the MS Society event. In general, we're lousy psychics. Let's get real about this: When we're worried about the future, it's because we're predicting that something awful will happen that has to do with either failure or rejection. These predictions can stick with us and continuously stress us out, because there's no end to the possibilities when you're imagining the future.

Being in other people's business. One of my favorite teachers, Byron Katie, says you must stay out of other people's business because you never know what other people are thinking or feeling. Ever. Even if they tell you, how do you know they're telling you the truth? Do *they* even know what they're really thinking? You can't be sure. This doesn't stop us from projecting what we think others will think or how they feel or how they will react. As with trying to predict the future, such predictions are almost never good. They usually involve imagining someone rejecting us or getting mad at us for something. That's stressful, but it's also voluntary, because we're choosing to worry about something that hasn't happened and may never happen, and that we truly have no idea about.

Arguing with reality. As Byron Katie says, "I'm a lover of reality. When I argue with what is, I lose, but only 100% of the time." There's no arguing with reality. What happens, happens. It's done. But we try to argue with it all the time anyway, like when we say something "shouldn't have happened" or that it "should be different," and by ruminating on it and getting stressed. "He shouldn't have said that. It made me feel like crap." Thinking that thought could make us feel mad or frustrated. There's usually a whole story behind why he shouldn't have said what he said, and how we would feel better if he hadn't said it at all. But what he said doesn't matter, because it's done. Arguing with reality is stressful because we will never win.

What do all of these categories of voluntary stress have in common? They're all thoughts. Most importantly, they're thoughts we can control, because we can choose what we believe.

Try It—Teasing It Out

When something is really bothering you, it's hard to simply say, "Oops—there goes my thinking. I'll just stop it now." But it is helpful to see if you can understand what thoughts you're having that are stressing you out.

Writing thoughts down can help. Once you have your thoughts in front of you on paper, it's easier to realize that nothing outside of you has to change for you to stop stressing out. And that's the best news ever, if you ask me.

Start with the Thought Storm exercise from Chapter 3—pick an issue that's stressing you out and do a thought storm about it—for three minutes, write out everything you think about the issue.

Go back over the list and separate the facts from the thoughts. This will show you what is reality and what is a thought about reality. Remember, reality doesn't make you mad or frustrated or happy. Reality is neutral. It's your subjective thoughts that carry the emotional charge. I find that even doing the first two parts of the exercise goes a long way toward helping me calm down when I'm upset.

Next to each thought, note whether or not it's about something that's in your control. For example, *He shouldn't have said that* is about something that's not in my control. On the other hand, the thought *I'm so mad at him* is about something that's within my control.

For each thought—both about things that are in your control and thoughts that aren't—ask yourself how that thought makes you feel; especially do this for the thoughts about factors you can't control. Ask yourself if those thoughts are serving you or your well-being. Are they helping you when you feel that way?

If they're not helping you, ask yourself if you can let those thoughts go.

Teasing It Out

....

What's stressing you out?

Write down all your thoughts about it. No editing, no correcting, no holds barred. (No one has to see this but you. The uglier the better.)

_____

_____

_____

_____

_____

_____

_____

_____

_____

_____

_____

_____

_____

_____

_____

_____

_____

_____

Go through what you just wrote—separate out the facts and thoughts by highlighting everything that is a thought.

Facts are objective and thoughts are subjective.

Teasing It Out (Part Two)

....

Write down each thought below.

Next to each thought, answer these questions:

How does each thought make you feel?

Is this thought serving you or holding you back? How?

Thought: _____

Emotion thought created: _____

Is this serving you or holding you back? How? _____

_____

_____

Thought: _____

Emotion thought created: _____

Is this serving you or holding you back? How? _____

_____

_____

Thought: _____

Emotion thought created: _____

Is this serving you or holding you back? How? _____

_____

_____

Thought: _____

Emotion thought created: _____

Is this serving you or holding you back? How? _____

_____

_____

GET YOUR OWN TEASING IT OUT SHEET!
Visit *www.AndreaHansonCoaching.com/BookSheets*
and download the free Teasing It Out worksheet
with added bonus questions.

I'll run you through an example of doing this Teasing It Out exercise.

My client, Jessica, was stressed about how her mother would react to a conversation they were going to have. Jessica's thought storm was very to the point and included thoughts like: *Mom's irrational. She's going to scream at me. She'll overreact—she always does.* Jessica was also thinking, *My brother is never around. I always have to do this. He should have to deal with this sometimes, too. He avoids this conversation on purpose.*

First, we separated out these facts: She will talk to her mother. She will bring up what she wants to talk about. Her brother will not be there.

Then we looked at Jessica's thoughts: *Mom's irrational. She's going to scream at me. She'll overeact. My brother is never around. I always have to do this. He avoids this conversation on purpose.*

When Jessica looked at her list of thoughts, she saw examples of arguing with reality and of being in her mother's and her brother's business. All of her thoughts were stressful and none of them were true—because they were sweeping generalizations, opinions, or predictions.

When she looked at her list of thoughts, something happened that often does when we write out thoughts and study them. Jessica saw her thoughts as just thoughts. She saw that they weren't true, and she saw how each one made her stress out about the upcoming conversation with her mother.

At that point, she was willing to let them go.

Jessica didn't force herself to believe something different. She simply realized that the thoughts she'd been thinking weren't true and weren't serving her. Letting go of those thoughts was possible because she came to realize there were other ways to look at the situation. She saw that her thoughts were not reality and they didn't serve her going forward.

So she released them.

Then she decided how she *wanted* to feel when she spoke with her mother. Not only was she able to meet with her mother without the stress, she was also able to reach a calm resolution with her mother, one that would not have been likely if Jessica had begun the conversation with her mother while she was stressed out by all those unobserved and unquestioned thoughts.

Putting It All Together

Worries can become very big and consume our attention. One thing leads to the next and our predictions about what's going to happen quickly spiral downward. If we're not paying attention, we come to believe a long list of thoughts and consequences that "prove" we will become helpless.

But when we list out our thoughts on paper, they take on a different form. Sometimes we see their ridiculousness right away. A common reaction once thoughts are on paper is, "Seriously? I can't believe I was even thinking that!" We're also more likely to notice the reality of the situation. And reality itself—no matter what it is—is never stressful. Our thoughts about reality are what stress us out.

Reducing voluntary stress is about seeing thoughts as just thoughts, and making informed decisions about whether to keep them or not.

We are not our thoughts. But our thoughts do trigger our emotions, so our thoughts cause how we feel. When thoughts stay in our heads unobserved they seem very real and feeling better seems impossible. But if we write our thoughts down, we can separate who we are from what we think. That's when we can start to see that those thoughts aren't as real as we once believed and we can say, "No, thank you," to our thoughts that cause pain.

What are you worried about right now? What tends to stress you out? What currently riles you up that you wish you could remain calm about? What do you rant about? What do you want to change?

Whatever stresses you out, you have the ability to feel better about it. However you want to feel instead of stress is possible. The only real control we have in life is over how we think and feel about things. We can use that control without being very aware of it and keep our stress levels high, or we can use that control to bring stress down and improve our health—and our sanity. That's a tremendous amount of power to have.

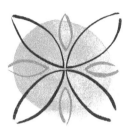

Chapter 6

Be Extraordinary to Yourself

What if you were in a relationship with someone who was constantly putting you down? Calling you fat, lazy, ugly, and stupid. Accusing you of not trying hard enough or not doing the right things. Never acknowledging your accomplishments, or how hard you're trying. And pouring salt in your wounds when you failed.

What if you could never get away from this person? What if they were always in your ear, interrupting your concentration? Butting in, and ruining all your happy moments?

What if this person kept you from setting big goals because she said you would never succeed? What if they were crafty about it, telling you all these things in a kind, I'm-just-looking-out-for-you voice, and yet however nice and rational their tones, you still felt guilty, upset, discouraged, alone, and tired?

Wouldn't you want out of that relationship?

I was in a relationship exactly like that one for most of my life. I felt exhausted and insecure all the time. But no other person was doling out the insults. There was no one for me to retaliate against, or to blame for how bad I felt.

Because that person was *me*.

Unveiling Myself

As I started practicing awareness of what I was thinking and feeling, and looking at where my stress was coming from, I unveiled a blatant truth: I was a total nightmare to myself. My relationship with myself was heinous. I was apathetic, manipulative, and downright brutal. I bullied myself. I lied to myself. I was a master of creating situations where I was damned if I did and damned if I didn't.

The more aware of my thoughts I became, the more I saw what was going on. I was truly taken aback by how often I was beating myself up. I became sad about the way I was treating myself. I would never, ever, say such mean things to someone else. But saying them to myself was apparently fine.

I'm not alone in acting this way. As we become more aware of the thoughts in our heads, we may notice that many of them are self-deprecating. When we become aware that what we think causes how we feel, it becomes more obvious that we are the instigators of our own negative feelings.

Why do we do this to ourselves?

We want what's best for us. We crave that ideal life, the one that often looks like being healthy and happy with a six-figure job and a closet full of size two clothes.

But somehow, sometimes, in the quest for well-being, we decide that scare tactics and threats are what will get the job done. We think we're being helpful and motivating. We think we'll stay on the couch eating ice cream all day unless we're hard on ourselves. We call this *getting serious about change* and *tough love*. We think we're saving ourselves from self-destruction.

The truth is, we don't need to be saved from anything.

What Creates Such Bad Behavior?

There are a few reasons why we lovingly think we need a constant ass-kicking. First, scare tactics are a part of the job description for a specific area of our brain. This area of our brain wants us to stay in a safe little hole far away from any risky behavior. Some call this the Lizard Brain, others call it the Monkey Mind, and it's commonly known as the "fight, flight, or freeze" response. The scientific name for this is the *amygdala*, and it has done a very good job for thousands of years of pointing out dangers and creating effective fear responses to keep humans alive.

This ancient part of the brain wants us to stay with the pack, be unnoticed, and keep away from danger. But now that we humans don't travel in packs so much and there are fewer sabertoothed tigers roaming around, the amygdala isn't needed on a daily basis to keep us physically safe. That doesn't stop it from speaking up when we want to change something. To the Lizard Brain, anything that looks different from the status quo is risky. Change could mean danger.

The Lizard Brain controls the voice that says we will fail miserably if we go for it. We'll make fools of ourselves and be rejected by other people if we try something new. It's the part that pokes fun at what we're doing in an effort to get us to stop doing it and crawl back into that safe hole. It's mean and scary, and it's the reason all our future projections lead to theoretical bag lady-dom. And yet, we are in control of that voice. We can tell it, "Thank you, but you're not helping."

The second reason we are so mean to ourselves is that the unattended mind honestly thinks criticism is helping to keep us motivated. I've spoken to many people who are convinced they wouldn't be motivated to work out if they didn't grab a handful of their fat and remark on how gross it is. The only problem is that if they really paid attention to what they're doing, they'd realize they feel awful about themselves and, as a result, they don't stick with working out for very long. We may think this is a constructive way to push ourselves farther and accomplish more, but it actually demotivates us, creating a struggle before we even start moving our bodies.

I use the term *unattended mind* because when we first start becoming aware of our thoughts, we often notice a big rush of nastiness. The unattended mind would rather you not notice it. Our minds have good intentions. They just need a little direction, which is what we give them, once we've taken a look and seen what's really going on in there.

When I first noticed the bullying I was dishing out to myself, I got really mad. It all seemed very contradictory and unhelpful. Bullying myself kept me from new accomplishments and kept me from truly shining. At first, when I noticed myself saying something mean to myself, I would respond by saying, "That's not nice!" And I would try not to think the mean thought again. But I soon noticed that my reactions held me in the same patterns, because I was bullying the bully. That doesn't work on the playground at school and it won't work in the playground of our minds, either.

Your Own Personal Browbeating

It's important to observe how self-bullying looks for you. What are your hot buttons? For some people, the buttons are around their weight and trying to get healthier. For others, the hot buttons may be about family or job performance.

What sets you off on a self-bullying tirade?

When we're mean, it isn't always through an overt comment. *You will never be able to do this!* Well, that thought is obviously mean, and so it's easy to spot. But thoughts can be sneaky.

One way I was being mean to myself was by thinking, *It is what it is*. I thought this was helping me recognize a fact. I thought I was being logical and accepting of reality. But when I took a closer look, I discovered a few things that surprised me.

First, when I really paid attention, I noticed that *It is what it is* made me feel a little depressed and hopeless. I was telling myself there was nothing I could do about the situation. Remember that a major sign that you're stating a fact is that you don't feel emotional about it. *That car is red. I own a laptop.* I feel nothing when I think those thoughts. But when I thought *It is what it is* I felt a twinge of hopelessness. Feeling emotion is a sign that what I'm looking at is a subjective thought or an opinion, rather than a fact.

When I thought *It is what it is*, what I meant was I thought there wasn't anything I could do to change the situation. But, often, that's not true at all.

Thoughts can be pervasive, and a thought like *It is what it is* may not stay isolated, affecting only one subject. When we truly believe something, we can apply the belief to many different issues. Bad haircut? *It is what it is*. Missed appointment? *It is what it is*. Spilled milk? *It is what it is*. You can see how it quickly a thought becomes a pattern, often without us noticing it's happening. And then believing this thought limits the range of responses we might have to anything and everything.

The time I most used *It is what it is* was when I was first diagnosed. It helped me reconcile myself to having MS and not worry about how I got it. But I realized very quickly that MS isn't *what it is*, because I have so much influence over my MS and my overall wellness.

Try It—What Are Your Mean Thoughts?

How do *you* beat yourself up?

Many bullying thoughts are glaring, like when one of my clients called herself fat on a daily basis. Some thoughts are a little sneakier. Maybe you tell yourself *It doesn't matter* if you do something you know isn't serving you, like eating a food you know you're allergic to. Some thoughts sound like constructive criticism, but are really only rudeness, like *That sounds stupid* or *Everyone will laugh.*

The way to start changing your thoughts is to get really curious and observe how you talk to yourself. I often have my clients keep a thought log for one week, writing down every bullying thought they have. The litmus test is how each thought makes you feel. If you feel beaten down, upset, like a failure, or you want to hide, your thought is mean.

Examples of common meanies are:

- *Whatever. It doesn't matter.*
- *I have to. I have no choice.*
- *I don't care.*
- *I shouldn't be taking this break.*
- *I'm not as good/skinny/likeable as they are.*
- *No one listens to me.*
- *Why can't I just stop?*

Often there are about 15 main offenders, mean thoughts that we think over and over. Remember those channels that form in our brains when we truly believe something and think it often? Some of those brain channels are for thoughts like *I'm lazy* or *Nothing I do will matter.* Pay attention for a week to find out how you're talking to yourself.

Another good test to see whether a thought is mean or not is to ask yourself if you would talk to a friend that way. Often we wouldn't dare.

While you're becoming aware of your thoughts, it's important not to judge yourself or get mad if you come across super-mean thoughts. Just notice.

Your Inner Meany

....

We're often hard on ourselves, but we don't realize that it's not helpful. It can cause demotivation, procrastination and zap our energy.

Notice for one week what mean thoughts you direct toward yourself. Start the list here:

_____

_____

_____

_____

_____

_____

_____

_____

_____

_____

_____

_____

_____

_____

_____

Do you notice repeat offenders? Are there thoughts that you often think in different situations?

_____

_____

_____

HAVE YOU DOWNLOADED YOUR FREE WORKSHEETS YET?

For an easy way to keep track of Your Inner Meany and other exercises in this book (plus bonus questions) go to *www.AndreaHansonCoaching.com/BookSheets*

The Bully Effect

My client, Ruby, needed to do physical therapy exercises every day. The exercises were personalized to her needs and helped her recuperate after a symptom flare-up. She knew the exercises were important, and they only took about ten minutes a day to complete, yet she wasn't doing them. She gave herself excuses like, "I don't have a good area in my house to do this." Or the all-encompassing justification, "I don't have time." Weeks would pass, and she still neglected her exercises.

When I asked Ruby why she wasn't doing her physical therapy, she said it was hard and she didn't feel good when she did it. She said she forgot about it. She said she didn't really know how to do it. She was the first to admit those were all easily solved issues.

When we talked about what she thought about her physical therapy, Ruby realized that the real problem was her thought that doing physical therapy meant she wasn't normal. "Normal people don't have to do this," she claimed. "Normal people can just walk without thinking about it. I'm supposed to do the exercises because I'm not like a normal person." She was telling herself that she no longer belonged to the "Normal Club." Her membership had been revoked when she got MS, and doing physical therapy was a glaring reminder. No wonder she wasn't doing her exercises!

If I was convinced that going to the mailbox meant I was abnormal, I would let my mail pile up. Ruby's thought that she wasn't allowed to be normal anymore was mean.

It's very common to think we're no longer normal once we get MS. But it's simply not true. When Ruby and I broke down what *normal* meant to her, she started to laugh because she realized there were probably only five people in the world who could meet her definition of normal.

She wasn't telling herself the truth with all those excuses. She was only being mean. But that mean thought was also stopping her from doing the valuable work to help herself.

After we broke down what Ruby thought about being normal, she was able to see that thinking she wasn't normal was what made her feel self-conscious and uninterested in doing her exercises. She didn't get mad at herself when she realized this. All she did was let her definition of *normal* go. She revised her thoughts to include the idea that doing her physical therapy meant she was getting better. She saw that the exercises were an important part of being kind to her body, and that doing physical therapy exercises didn't need to have anything to do with what other people thought of her.

Being mean to ourselves stops progress. I've looked, but I haven't found an upside to being mean to myself. If you consider self-bullying to be motivating, take a closer look. Even if you experience moments of motivation as a result of having mean thoughts about yourself, that motivation will be short-lived and making progress will be harder than it needs to be.

The Remedy

When I'm exploring this issue of mean self-thoughts with clients, I'm often asked how to "fix it." "If I know the self-bullying is happening, how can I fix it? How can I stop?" It's tempting to correct this pattern by simply trying not to be so mean. But consider how you would act if you said something mean to a friend. What if you said, "No one will like you if you do that," and then tried to change the subject? Would you really drop that mean bomb and then not even acknowledge what you'd just said afterward? Probably not. And if you did, it's not likely that you would be friends with that person for very long.

But you *are* a good friend. So chances are you'd stop, apologize for what you'd said, and let your friend know you didn't really intend to be rude. Maybe you'd even explain that you've got some big deadlines coming up at work and you're feeling stressed and so you spoke without thinking it through, and you regret it. You'd make an effort to say something truly constructive about what she's wanting to do, something that would help her improve her situation and feel good about herself.

We can do this with ourselves as well.

When you catch yourself thinking one of those bullying thoughts, stop and acknowledge it. If we sweep those thoughts under the rug, they're free to pop back up. When we really expose our thoughts and clean them up, there's less chance that they will make as much mess the next time. So don't deflect that thought. Carefully look at it instead. Why did you think it? What do you actually want to happen? What do you really want to do? What are you afraid of? Get to the root of *why* you had that bullying thought. There's a reason you thought it. Understanding that reason will move you to a deeper understanding of yourself and help you become truly motivated and productive.

Always Bring Kindness

As you go through the exercise above (and all the exercises in this book), bring your kindness with you. If you notice you're feeling upset and realize it's because of your own thinking, try not to be discouraged. As we get to know ourselves better, we may find things we don't like. I often say that if we don't find anything about ourselves that makes us cringe, we haven't looked hard enough. Those things will be there, and that's ok. You're looking at them now in order to clean them up and move them out. The way out of being mean to yourself is through kindness.

When I started focusing on how hard I was being on myself, the first thing I noticed was how often it happened. The second thing I noticed was that I gained a mountain of energy when I stopped.

Remember that person who constantly looks over your shoulder, comments on what you're doing, how you're doing it, and how bad your efforts are? Imagine that person saying all of those things with an "I told you so" inflection in their voice, too. Oh, and did I mention they're *always* around? You can never shake them.

Hanging out with a person like that might be a tiny bit draining. Especially if you're scrambling to please her, which you never can. It's exhausting.

When I got rid of the heckler looking over my shoulder I felt like I'd lost 20 pounds. I had crazy new energy and felt like I even had more time on my hands. Bullying, and the ensuing battle of wills, takes time and energy away from your day. Being kind takes way less focus and makes life a lot easier.

Do I ever rebound back to my former nightmare self? You bet. Old thoughts do pop back up. But I have them on security alert. I'm onto them, and onto myself. And so I apologize to myself, try to understand why I'm thinking the mean thought, and I move on, having given myself a mental hug.

When you take a look at your own thinking and behavior, see if you can pin down your self-bullying cues. Maybe you notice, as Ruby did, that you're *not* doing something that you know is important, and that alerts you to pause and eavesdrop on what you're thinking about it. Maybe a bullying thought shows up as procrastination. One of my cues to self-bullying is when I notice myself taking an extra long look at the cheesy poofs aisle at the grocery store and considering a reality TV marathon. When that happens, I know there's a reason I'm hiding behind fake food and fake TV, and the culprit is always my inner bully.

Get to know your bully so you can use kindness to send it on it's way. This is essential for keeping the peace in your head, and for reclaiming loads of energy in your mind and body. Then you can accomplish what's really important to you, while leaving the drama behind.

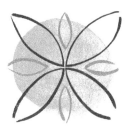

Chapter 7

How to Cultivate Energy

When I was first diagnosed with MS, I received big warnings about fatigue from people in the MS community. Their assumption that I had a problem with it was so often made without any inquiry about whether it actually affected me. "Just don't do too much at once," I was cautioned.

Those early warnings helped me realize that MS is very personal. Here were people telling me something *should* happen when, in actuality, it wasn't happening. If this was going on for me, I knew it was also going on for other people newly diagnosed with MS.

I'm willing to say that fatigue can be common for people living with MS. But I won't give you the statistics. No statistic will tell you if *you*, personally, will experience fatigue, or to what extent it may be a problem. Getting connected with yourself and what is really happening in your body will.

How much and how easily you feel MS-related fatigue is completely individual. I've had MS for over 15 years, and not once have I experienced the *running through molasses* feeling of MS fatigue. If I had accepted the statistics, I would have spent more than 15 years waiting and watching for fatigue and thinking about it. Whenever I got tired, I would have wondered, "Is that MS?" Eventually, I would have believed it was.

The Human Factor

Energy is one of the most important commodities we have. Learning to cultivate energy is an important aspect of connecting with our bodies and learning what we personally need. I have a whole section on cultivating energy in the program I teach, because I've discovered we often do things to rob ourselves of this precious resource.

Although guarding energy is especially important when you have MS, it's important even if you don't have the diagnosis. In this chapter, I point out factors that rob anyone of energy, not only people with MS or with MS-related fatigue.

When I think about my energy, I don't tell myself, *I have to be careful because I have MS.* I just say, *It's a human thing to care about my energy levels. We all should do it.* I think this is important because it removes that daily reminder of *I have MS* and replaces it with *I'm just human.*

Because energy is so personal, everyone has her own cocktail of actions that sap energy and that bring it back. Let's look at a few of the major energy-killers. They're the usual suspects, the things that make us collapse at the end of the day (with true MS fatigue and/or because we're human) if we don't get enough of them.

Sleep

This seems obvious. To have energy, you need enough sleep. You know you're a different person when you get quality sleep. I hear from a lot of people that they don't sleep well, for various reasons. It's worth paying attention to sleep quality, because sleep is a wonder drug. A chronic lack of it should not be taken lightly. Sleep provides you with energy, but it also helps you process your day and your emotions, and helps with cognitive functioning.

Sleep can be complicated. I look at the issue of getting enough sleep as multi-faceted. The first thing to do to nurture your energy is optimize your sleep situation.

Here's a rundown of things you can do on our own: Plan for eight hours of sleep (or however many hours you need for true rejuvenation) and make sure the bed, pillow, and covers are right for you. Make sure you're in complete darkness, and make the room temperature colder. If you're like me and have a dog, give her a separate place to sleep so she won't bother you. I know we love our fur babies, but if they constantly wake us up at night, game over. This is no time to mess around. Turn off or cover up those little blue lights on electronics in the bedroom and avoid watching TV and reading anything that's backlit for a while before going to sleep. Another factor than can be overlooked are blood sugar levels. If you fall asleep easily but wake up in the early hours of the morning, your blood sugar may be dropping at night and waking you up. Talk with a holistic professional to get more insight.

Doing some of these things may mean changing your routine, which can mean some internal protest. If you find yourself defending the fact that you can only fall sleep with the TV on in the background, ask yourself one question: What means more to you—your long-term health or half-watching bad late night TV that you won't even remember in a week? To get a good night's sleep, I changed quite a bit of my nightly ritual, with protests in tow. Now I defend my sleep optimization like it's worth a million dollars. To me, it is.

There is a next level of sleep optimization. If you've tried everything and are still having problems getting enough sleep, know that you are worth calling in the big guns. Talk to your doctor about your medication's side effects. See if there's another prescription that would help. Even go to a sleep doctor and have a sleep study done.

You and your sleep are worth the fuss.

Hydration

Julia had to postpone a coaching session with me for a few days because she needed to recoup after becoming fatigued. She had helped a good friend for almost 14 hours straight, even though she knew she was pushing her limits. "After all," she reasoned, "I'm a loyal friend and that's what loyal friends do. "

"Did you drink water at all during that long day?" I asked. Julia was surprised by the question, but when she went back over the day, she realized she hadn't had any water at all. She'd allowed herself to become completely dehydrated. Julia experienced MS fatigue, but becoming dehydrated compounded it. Drinking plenty of water the next day helped her recuperate.

I've noticed that for my own cultivation of energy, staying hydrated is very important. When I'm dehydrated, I feel heavy and I don't want to do anything. My pep is totally gone.

Think about the last time you were dehydrated. How did it feel for you? My guess is that your energy took a hit. The good news is that your energy will rebound when you rehydrate.

Relaxation

One of the most surprising factors in cultivating energy comes from thinking. Or, technically, *not* thinking. Thinking about problems and being really hard on ourselves depletes energy without us moving a muscle. Real energy is spent when we ruminate on something that stresses us out or when we're caught in a shame cycle, being super-critical towards ourselves.

A pleasant surprise came when I started being kind to myself and paying attention to my thoughts. I gained so much energy that I almost didn't know what to do with it. I certainly had a lot of extra time and physical and mental energy, since I wasn't spending it on draining, cyclical thinking.

Exercise

Of course, one of the many benefits of exercise is increased energy. But have you ever had a great workout on a Saturday morning, pushed yourself to the limit, and then stayed on the couch watching TV for the rest of the day? If you push too much in your workouts, you'll be spent for the rest of the day. But if you know your sweet spot, working out can give you energy for the whole day. When you do this consistently, it improves basic health levels, like resting heart rate and blood pressure, and naturally puts you on a higher level of everyday energy.

Thinking We're Super Human

Leigh was at a conference that took place over a large campus. She was walking constantly, lugging her notebooks and laptop from room to room over multiple days of meetings. By the end of the conference, she was wiped out, beyond done. Her energy was spent and she needed a few days to recoup. When we first talked about it, she was somewhat surprised that she'd gotten so tired. She knew she'd walked a lot, and it had been a long couple of days, but to her the exhaustion seemed a little "all of a sudden."

Our willpower is mighty. We can keep going, doing what we feel we have to do, ignoring our cues to slow down in order to accomplish our goals. But, MS or not, there's a price to pay for doing that. Always.

I took Leigh though an exercise I call the Energy Timeline. By breaking down the three days of the conference, looking more carefully at each day, Leigh was able to pinpoint and become more aware of her different levels of energy and see how she reacted to each one during the conference.

When the conference started, Leigh felt great. She went to her meetings and walked all over the campus. As time wore on, she got more and more tired, but she didn't do anything about it. She pushed herself onward.

When she looked at why she kept pushing, she realized it was because she didn't want people to know she had MS and she thought that resting would clue them in. However, by acting like she didn't have MS, she pushed herself beyond what many of her colleagues (none of whom had MS) were able to do easily. She walked farther, carried more than she needed to, and didn't take enough breaks. She admitted she felt that she had something to prove. And while proving it, she'd ignored what her body told her and kept going.

In an effort to prove something, we may go way overboard. We become this super-human who doesn't stop. Sometimes it serves us and sometimes it backfires in a big way. Leigh found her efforts backfiring.

In her session with me, we went backwards in time over the conference experience to learn how her body had been talking to her. I asked Leigh to explain how her body felt on the third day, at the very end of the conference. She said she felt very lethargic and had slept for a long time afterwards. I asked her to go backwards from there and remember how her body felt the morning of the third day. She said she felt like she hadn't gotten enough rest (even though she'd slept a good eight hours). It had been really hard to get up and go.

We went back farther in time to the night of the second day. She said her body had been very tired. When I asked what her body was telling her, she thought about it for a minute and said, "It was really tired, but I thought maybe getting a good night's sleep would work."

We looked farther back in time to the middle of the second day, and her body had felt a little lighter. We went even farther back and Leigh found that on the first night her body had felt great—light and energized, ready to go.

We had identified her two extremes. The first day, her body felt light and energized and ready to go. By the end of the third day, her body was screaming at her to stop. In going through the timeline backwards, she was able to see that her body whispered to her on the second day that she needed to slow down and recoup her energy. Her body started to feel a bit heavier, even pulling her back. But she didn't listen, because she wasn't looking for the signs. By the end of the conference she was a surprised she was so tired.

Bringing It Back

Leigh learned something valuable. She learned how her body feels when it's giving her that light tap, tap, tap and saying, "Excuse me. I need more energy now, please."

We came up with quite a few personal strategies that would allow Leigh to give her body what it needed to keep going and remain energized. She could literally lighten her load by carrying only what she needed, she could increase her hydration, and she could simply slow down as she walked. She stopped trying to prove herself by going farther and faster than everyone else, and just breathed more.

When you're trying to boost your energy, there will be many techniques that will work for you. One of my favorites is to drink a glass of cold-pressed veggie juice (with maybe ten percent fruit juice). That rush of nutrition gives me hours of pep.

A solution that's often suggested to boost energy is good, strong coffee. Although I do love my coffee, I don't recommend it as a go-to energy enhancer because, depending on what's in it, coffee can give you an artificial boost that makes you crash later. The goal is not to create an energy rollercoaster, but to keep your energy on an even keel throughout the day.

When you take ongoing action to cultivate more energy, and notice sooner when your levels are getting depleted, it won't take as much to get them back up. You can remedy the situation before getting to a point of being completely spent and needing three shots of espresso with a side of sugar hooked up to an IV.

Try It—Energy Timeline

Think about a time when you were exhausted. It might have been on a day you accomplished a million things and then crashed at the end of it. Start at the end of that day and remember how your body physically felt. (The body meditation is a great technique to use here to recapture that information). Get to know the details: Did your body feel light or heavy? Did you have a specific feeling in your shoulders, back, or stomach? What was your body telling you at the end of the day?

Move backward a few hours. How did your body feel in the afternoon? Get as specific as you can. Were you starting to feel a little slower? Were you thirsty or tired? Your answers will be completely unique to you, so be really curious about them.

Then go back a few more hours to mid-day. How did your body feel then? Go back a little further to mid-morning, then back again to recall how your body felt when you first started your day.

For each time period, think about how your body felt and what it was trying to tell you. What you'll discover are your body's subtle communications about your energy levels. This is just like paying attention to your body while exercising.

This exercise gives you invaluable information. Once you know your body's whispers about energy, you will hear them loud and clear—before the whispers become a yell.

Energy Timeline

....

Our body speaks to us during the day about our energy levels. Think about a day you've had recently when you were wiped out at the end.

Going backwards through your day in 3-4 hour increments, use the body meditation and explain how your body felt at different times of the day.

What was your body telling you each time? When could you have used an energy boost?

Time: _____ (Crash at end of day)

_____

_____

Time: _____ (4 hours earlier)

_____

_____

Time: _____ (4 hours earlier)

_____

_____

Time: _____ (4 hours earlier)

_____

_____

Time: _____ (Wake up)

_____

_____

FOR AN EASY WAY TO TRACK BACK THROUGH A DAY TO LEARN YOUR ENERGY CUES GO TO: *www.AndreaHansonCoaching.com/BookSheets* and download your free, easy-to-use worksheet with added bonus questions.

Caveat

I'm not saying you should stop whatever you're doing. I'm not saying you should be less productive during your day. I'm not saying you should slack off at work or leave the kids waiting in the carpool line. How much you do in any given day is completely up to you, of course. But when you know your body's cues about your energy levels, you have more options.

What the Energy Timeline exercise will tell you is how to read your body's cues as they happen, so you can cultivate your energy and keep going at whatever speed works for you. Maybe cultivating your energy simply means hydrating more often and getting more sleep. Maybe it means taking 15 minutes to unplug and meditate during lunch. Maybe it means tightening up the logistics of your day. It doesn't mean you have to stop doing things that are important to you and your life.

Paying attention to energy levels not only keeps us from getting to the point of being spent, it also allows us to be more productive by being smarter.

There are a couple of physical feelings in my body that I watch out for. These are my cues to stop pushing myself and take a break. When my body's whispering at me to get my attention, I feel a slight heaviness. It's a specific type of heavy that tells me my body is tugging on me to slow down for a bit. Napping is a personal favorite way of mine (and my hubby's) to boost energy. A few minutes of meditation, or a walk, are energy boosters for me as well.

When I'm really getting spent, I have a *burning the candle at both ends* feeling. This is when I'm so absorbed in something, like when I'm working on a project, that I push right past the whisper. This sensation feels like being separated from my body, and I notice my mental focus is not as sharp. This is more like a loud knock, and when I "hear" it, I know I need to stop what I'm doing and pick it back up the next day.

When I listen to the whisper, it takes a lot less to recoup than when I ignore the whisper until it turns into that loud knock. No matter where I am on that spectrum between whisper and knock, I no longer wait for the yell. I see that as dangerous territory for my health.

What are your warning signs? What does your body feel like when you need to cultivate more energy? What does your body feel like when you have your own *burning the candle at both ends* moment?

Paying attention to your energy is one of the most loving and compassionate things you can do for yourself. Many people think they're superhuman and end up hurting themselves when they discover they're not. By learning to take care of your energy, you're definitely ahead of the curve.

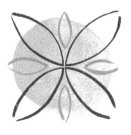

....

Chapter 8

....

The Truth About Honesty

Honesty can be tricky. When we're thinking about telling the truth to someone else, we can consider whether it's the friendly thing to do, whether it will hurt that person's feelings, and whether whatever it is we're thinking of saying needs to be pointed out at all. Sometimes it can be kinder to stay mum.

But what about when it comes to being honest with ourselves? Do we have the same considerations? What does it look like when we stay mum? We can't lie to ourselves because we see our own cards. When it comes to choosing what to say to ourselves, the opposite of honesty is denial.

Denial comes in different sizes. Sometimes it's blatantly ignoring the pink polka-dotted elephant in the room. But there are other, smaller types of denial that can also hurt. Like ignoring that inner voice that says the doughnut isn't healthy—or even wanted. Denial in this case is very small, just a bit of something we're not completely honest with ourselves about. But that softer side of denial can hurt as well. That's because denial in any amount creates a cache of stress that builds up over time.

Honesty on the other hand, relieves that stress. The honesty discussed here is with ourselves. It's ok if you're not ready to shout all your truths to the outside world. You don't have to. We can be honest with ourselves without letting anyone else know. This is personal.

Getting honest with myself has been a big source of energy, kindness, and stress relief. But achieving that honesty has also been one of the toughest things I've done.

Any area of your life is fair game when it comes to denial: MS, your weight, your finances, relationships, or anything else. The possibilities are endless. Each day brings something new to consider denying.

Denial can masquerade as the path of least resistance. There may be an area of your life that you know needs your attention, but when you look at it you feel uncomfortable. So you look the other way, toward something more pleasant. You think the discomfort will go away when you stop paying attention, but the issue you're in denial about is not what's painful. It's the denial itself that delivers all that discomfort.

When you stop paying attention to the issues, the bad feelings don't go away. They stick around in the form of dread, embarrassment, or fatigue. You can ignore the issue all you want, but it's tough to ignore being in denial about it.

Denial Is in the Details

When we're facing something big, it's tempting to only take a peek at first. Lift the covers a teensy bit and see the edge of what's out there. Then pull the covers back over our heads, thinking *I already knew that was there*, and tell ourselves we'll deal with it later.

We may feel like we're confronting the issue simply by not denying that it's there. We're taking medication and working out, so there's no denial about MS here, right? But that's the sneaky thing about denial—it can make us feel like we're doing something, when we're mostly looking the other way. We can deal quite well with the top layer while ignoring the bigger danger floating below the surface.

If denial is so sneaky, how do we know we're in it?

Maybe we get a nagging feeling when a topic is broached, and we don't want to read or even hear about that subject. We quickly say to ourselves, *That doesn't apply to me,* and hurry to focus on something else. We feel like we have a dirty little secret. If we think about that topic, we get restless, edgy, or snippy. We want to literally get up, run away, and/ or fight for our right to not see it as a problem.

From day one, I accepted that I had MS. Or so I thought. I immediately started drug therapy, working out, and openly talked about my diagnosis. During the first five years of my diagnosis, I would never have considered myself to be in denial, but I was. Anytime I heard a suggestion that something could go wrong with my MS, I became angry. Anytime someone assumed I had a "common" symptom of MS, I would shut him or her out mentally. If someone suggested my health could go downhill, I would label them as *not helpful,* and turn away. The people telling me that awful things would happen were often healthcare professionals and/or other people with MS. I would feel myself pushing them away. *They don't understand that what they're saying won't happen to me.* I thought I was helping and empowering myself when I turned away from people who thought I was going to fall apart. I thought I was protecting myself by pushing away negative influences.

But then I noticed that I had a nagging feeling and a quick-to-condemn reaction when anyone even asked me what my MS symptoms were. I became upset. *They made me go there.* Even though I fully admitted I had MS, I was still in denial about what could happen—and that wasn't beneficial. That denial kept me running and constantly on guard, ready to deflect anything I didn't deem helpful to hear.

It was my *reaction* to the attitudes people had about MS that wasn't helpful. My reaction had consumed me more than I realized, and had long ago passed the point of being protective. What hurt me wasn't what other people were saying. Others are going to have their own beliefs. I can't change that. What hurt me was my own resistance to their beliefs and opinions. That resistance, I discovered, wasn't born out of a desire to protect myself. It was born out of fear. I was in denial about how I really felt.

Be Confrontational

When it comes to denial, confrontation is truly the only way to end it. Denial is like an unwanted houseguest. It won't get the hints. If we try to be nice, it ignores us. Denial has moved in, is sleeping in our bed and using our toothbrush, and it's not going to leave without a direct confrontation.

The only way to make denial leave is to stand up for yourself and trust that you'll be ok if things get ugly. This is not an easy process, but getting out of the grip of denial will rock your world (in a good way).

I realized that in order to fully support my health, that edgy, nagging feeling of being in denial had to go. I decided to confront everything that scared me about having MS. I started looking head-on at the symptoms that could stop me, physically and cognitively. I told the truth to myself for the first time. I admitted I was terrified of defeat. I said out loud how daunted I was by the prospect of never recovering from a relapse. I choked on the words every time I talked about my deepest fears, and how this disease could make those fears a reality.

I realized that I couldn't stand hearing people who didn't know me say certain things would happen to me—because what if they were right? I didn't want to give them the satisfaction of knowing better than

I did what would happen to me. I was so afraid that opening up honestly about my fears would make every last one of them come true.

But I opened up anyway.

And as I was laying everything out, something amazing happened. I let the fears run through me. I let myself sit in the vulnerability of *what could happen*. And then a light bulb went on. I realized that none of the circumstances I feared were actually happening. *What if* wasn't the same as *what is*. My fear was of a future that hadn't occurred. And even if it did happen, I realized clearly that it wouldn't devastate me. I would deal with it.

When I pushed through my denial and flushed my fears out from their hiding place, I saw that my fears weren't real. I had done a great job of convincing myself that they were real, because I'd thought I had lots of logical evidence, but it didn't hold up once I shone the light of honesty on it.

I later learned from Brené Brown, renowned researcher and author of *Daring Greatly*, that fear and denial thrive in the dark, but fall apart when you hold them up to the light for scrutiny. When I denied my fears, they didn't go anywhere. They remained, shut away in the dark, unspoken, rising up again whenever someone told me about my future with MS.

Being Honest Is Crucial

It's easy to assume the truth will hurt. But what hurts us the most is fearing the truth and lying to ourselves. Especially when we think it's only a little white lie that's doing us the favor or distracting us from what's really happening.

There's relief in honesty. Even if we're being honest about something big and scary, it feels so good to let go of the lie and own that we're afraid. Because then something different can happen.

Honesty takes courage.

As I began paying attention to my thoughts, I was tempted to be less than honest with myself about everything, because reality often wasn't pretty and positive. I thought speaking the negative thoughts would hurt me. We have to be willing look at all the ugly bits to create our best health possible. The hardest part of banishing denial is often stepping into the willingness to look. When we do, quite often we find that the ugly bits aren't so ugly.

When we're honest with what we're thinking and how we're really feeling, we can better see the places that need attention. We can better understand how we really want to feel. We can see the discrepancies and close the gaps.

Honesty about our stress and energy levels and how we're physically feeling allows us to see ourselves more clearly. That can be liberating. We start to feel even more comfortable with telling ourselves the truth. That comfort gives us permission to acknowledge the little changes we notice in our bodies, and it positions us to address those little changes before they become big flare-ups.

Being honest with yourself is the foundation of living a healthy life.

When I was honest with myself about my fears, the way I looked at my world changed. It became clear that the blanket, negative predictions that threatened me and triggered my denial never came from my neurologist or from the people in my inner circle. They came from people who were one step removed from the people and the opinions I trusted. So I tightened my list of advisors (doctors, coaches, and other healers) to include only those who know me personally and who also listen to me before assuming they know about me.

I also began to have a different reaction when someone told me something bad would happen to me. It no longer hurt. No matter who was predicting something bad for me—a health care professional, an organization, another person with MS—I came to realize that what they said wasn't personal.

What I began to realize was that these were other people's own fears about MS. What they'd seen had scared them, and they wanted someone to be scared with. With that perspective, I even found that I could lovingly hear their fears and know that what they said had nothing to do with me.

Sympathy helps when dealing with something new, like the initial blow that comes with a diagnosis. But constant sympathy coming toward us, and continuously sharing our fears with others, doesn't help us move forward. In some cases, it keeps us stuck. To feel better, we need to be honest about what we're afraid of—and simply feel the emotion for those 90 seconds or so until the feeling dissipates. It takes courage and a willingness to be vulnerable, but it can be so worth it.

I don't know what my future holds, but neither does anyone else. I no longer carry resistance and anger toward people who try to tell me what will happen to me. Instead, I've found love and compassion for what they're going through. Letting go of the pain that came from taking on other people's fears as my own, or from staying in denial, was an important healing experience for me.

Knowing Your Tell

A "tell" is a behavior that shows up when someone is bluffing, like while playing poker. You may have a certain facial expression, a subtle tic, or an obvious look. *There's nothing to see here.* Rookie poker players may not pick up on others' or even their own tells, but professionals can often see tells from a mile away. Knowing your competitor's tells can give you an advantage in the card game. Knowing your own tells can help you secure a win.

There are many ways to bluff about the things going on in our lives—about anything from our finances to our relationships to our health. We can bluff about whether we can afford a new car, when in actuality our finances are in the red every month. We can bluff that we're really happy in a relationship and consider it fine that we fight all the time. We can bluff that we're taking the best care of our health, while ignoring a gut feeling that something's wrong. Bluffing goes both ways. We can have great health and still bluff, as I did, by assuming we need to fear that something will go wrong any minute.

What are your tells when you're bluffing? Often a tell is something we find ourselves saying. For example, thinking *I already knew that* can be a tell. We may say it because we truly do already know and understand. But *I already knew that* is also a deflection statement. When you already know something and turn away, you push away the possibility of finding out more, telling yourself you don't need to. But what if you do? What might you find if you stayed open?

Bluffing shows up in excuses, like when we don't say what we're really thinking. Where do you make excuses instead of telling yourself or someone else the whole truth?

Another way to uncover a tell is by paying attention to how we feel emotionally. It hurts when we're not totally honest. There can be a twinge of anger that comes up because we don't want to think about something. What does that twinge feel like for you?

A non-subtle tell is when we get defensive. We may push back, even forcefully, at a subject when we don't want to admit something. Maybe we don't want to admit that we're wrong or that there's another way to look at an issue. Whatever it is, we want nothing to do with it. Defensiveness was my tell. It came to a head when I didn't want to hear what could go wrong with my MS. That was my cue to take a look at why I was being so defensive. Defensiveness is like a door that opens us up to the exact point of our fears. What topics or situations do you find yourself being defensive around?

We can bluff in any area of our lives. Your biggest bluff right now may not be about MS at all, but something seemingly unrelated, like your relationship with your child or your job. Tells don't happen in isolation. Nor do bluffs. Just like our thoughts, they tend to show up in patterns. The specifics of what you're bluffing about don't matter as much as understanding your particular tell. Because your tell acts as a beacon, indicating exactly where you can find denial in any part of your life. Once you know where your denial is, you can choose to face it head on.

What's your tell? Is it a feeling in your gut, a habit of physically walking away, or a phrase you repeat? Everyone has tells. With a little sleuthing, you can find yours and use it to bring more healing honesty into your life.

Try It—Finding the Needle in a Haystack

Looking for places you're being less than honest with yourself can feel like finding a needle in a haystack. How can you find denial when it's so sneaky, when we're so good at covering things up when we don't want to face them? How do you know whether or not you're in denial if you're feeling like you're completely honest with yourself and like nothing needs to change?

When we *decide* to be honest with ourselves, we begin to see where we're not being honest. It's simple, but not easy. It starts with that decision, that vow of deciding to find the courage to see what you previously didn't want to see.

Give yourself one week of honesty, even if you feel like you're already always honest. No matter how ugly it gets, tell yourself the truth. Instead of thinking, *This ice cream won't hurt me*, you might realize the truth is more like *I like ice cream and am willing to take the consequences because it's tasty*. Admitting that may feel silly at first, but if that's the truth, it's going to feel better and help you more.

Give yourself the respect you deserve. Be honest about why you're doing things. Most importantly, show yourself compassion when you admit your truths, which may be contradictory and messy. They will also be enlightening.

Be kind to yourself as you engage in this process.

If you do this for one week, you'll likely notice a pattern of telling yourself some little white lies. You'll also likely notice when you're using excuses, which may be while you're on autopilot and not paying attention to your thoughts. Start to examine those patterns and chances are they'll reveal something you're bluffing about.

Be Brave

No matter what part of your life you examine, bravery is an essential part of eliminating denial. When you uncover an area you've been in denial about and really see the truth, the whole landscape of your life will be affected. Once you see how diving into one area splashes everything else, the process can get uncomfortable. This is tough work at first. It calls for a lot of faith—first, that you're doing what's best for you, and ultimately that there's a way through. Immense and wonderful things can happen when you completely back out of your denial state and see the picture of your life in full daylight.

Keep moving forward. Pulling the blinders back over your eyes is no longer an option. Your momentum and the vision of what you want your health and your life to look like will likely sharpen your resolve and bring new awareness. For instance, you may begin to receive more assistance in creating your new reality from people and resources you hadn't known existed. Circumstances will tend to come together in just the right way to give you boosts along your journey. Swift solutions will become more common. That swiftness comes when you flip the switch from resisting what's happening to allowing it and facing it with conviction. Instead of turning your back and running away, you start running toward what you fear—and the game switches from chase to chicken.

And you, my friend, are not the chicken.

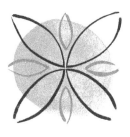

Chapter 9

Putting the Layers Together

My neurologist gave me valuable advice the first week I was diagnosed with MS. He said there would be a lot of alternative therapies suggested to me and I should be careful about what I try. He was in no way trying to warn me off of treatments—he was letting me know there are strong opinions out there about how MS should be treated.

Alternative therapy is treatment outside of traditional drug therapy. Someone using only dietary changes and not taking traditional medication is using an alternative therapy approach. *Complementary therapy* is when an alternative treatment is done in conjunction with a traditional drug therapy. Someone who is implementing dietary changes while taking traditional drug therapy is using a complementary therapy approach.

The majority of people living with MS use a complementary therapy approach.

I have found that most people who suggest specific alternative therapies seem to do so out of the goodness of their hearts. I choose to think that everyone genuinely wants to help, and believes in his or her solution. If only sincere enthusiasm was all we needed to know if something works. But it's not.

I learned pretty soon after my diagnosis that it's good to vet therapies for ourselves so we know if they work for us. Even if it's a traditional drug therapy that works for thousands, we still need to do our own research. Every time.

Deciding on a diet to follow, now that you have MS, is a great example of why it's helpful to research and figure out what works for you personally. What we eat can be a layer containing multiple variables. Later in this chapter, I'll talk about how all the layers fit together. First, I want to talk more specifically about food. Many people want to know, "Is there a diet that can help my MS?" It can seem like a new diet is recommended each week for us to try, which can leave us confused and overwhelmed about what feels like a crucial choice.

The Dietary Layer

Diet is a very important part of staying healthy. To clarify, when I say *diet* I mean *the food we eat*. This is not about cutting calories to get skinny, but about choosing food and nutrients that nourish our bodies. There are a number of diets that claim to help people with MS. These diets can generally be put into one of two categories: paleo-based or macrobiotic-based. Many of these diets are backed by scientific studies and/or by people with MS who say that diet has helped them immensely, and even cured them of symptoms. I love that we have helpful books and programs that make eating easy for us. The problem is that these two categories of diets, both with supporters claiming they help MS, are very different from each other.

One says whole grains are good, the other says gluten is the devil. One says beans and starches are great, the other says to stay away from anything starchy and white. One recommends large portions of meat and natural fats, the other recommends very small portions of anything from an animal. How can diets from both categories have testimonials from people saying their diet works for and even cures MS?

Because all of those diets are right. For some people.

There are also other diets, ones that haven't (yet) been as scientifically studied or proven to be effective for some people with MS, and they may be right as well. This is because whether a diet works or not depends on the individual more than the diet.

Some specifics remain the same across all the diets I've seen that are said to be good for people with MS (and good for humans in general): organic foods, cutting back on sugar, cutting out preservatives completely, eating food that's as natural as possible, and eating large portions of fresh vegetables and some fruit. The common recommendation is to eat foods that are as whole as possible, which means foods that are minimally processed. For example, eat an apple instead of pre-packaged applesauce.

I have personally heard many stories from people who say they significantly improved their body's reactions to MS by changing their diet. Health with MS is not simply about eliminating food groups, but finding what you body needs. The end goal is to heal our bodies with food choices, not to create mass deficits of nutrients. As I discuss in my book, *Stop Carrying the Weight of Your MS*, the key is to figure out on our own what specific diet works for us. To clarify, we should still get data and expertise from sources we trust, but you and your body are the final decision makers for what ultimately works for you. What works for you may be the exact replica of a diet that works for someone else, it may be a mash-up of aspects of a few diets, or it may be a way of eating you put together on your own from what feels good and works for your body.

When diagnosed with MS, many of us try going gluten-free. I did. Many times. I felt better each time I tried again to eat gluten-free, but I also noticed a few crucial things. First, I could eat a little wheat here and there and nothing bad would happen—it didn't make me feel lethargic or upset my digestion. So I figured I wasn't massively allergic to gluten, but only a little bit intolerant. Then I had three different, conclusive tests done (I'm nothing if not thorough) and they all said I don't have Celiac Disease. Also, I never felt *awesome* when I stopped eating gluten, only a little better. My body was whispering to me that something else in my diet might be having more of an impact.

I turned to an allergist for help with my quest and had more tests done. The results confirmed that my body is not allergic to wheat or gluten (unless the gluten is in isolation, which it rarely is). My body is allergic to corn. What grain had I been eating to replace wheat? Corn. When I stopped eating corn, I *did* feel awesome. Staying corn-free is easy for me, because there's no question that my body feels better when I go without it.

Some proponents of diets for improving health for people with MS say that corn is ok to eat, while others say it's not. Taking the time to notice how my body reacted to each dietary change I made, instead of blindly following an entire diet, was crucial for figuring what really worked for me and what didn't.

Be mindful of the diets and therapies you choose, instead of going with what the experts advise without first confirming that it works for you.

It Can Be Complicated

This book is not about providing a one-size-fits-all approach. I wish healing were that easy. Even if we have the same diagnosis of MS, we are not the same. We have different genes and backgrounds and we've experienced different environments. We have different routines and habits. We may even have different types of MS.

Because of all those differences, different therapies will work for each of us.

Scientists still don't know what causes any of the forms of MS. What they do know is that part of the cause lies in dozens of our genes, and gene variations can vary depending on our environment.

In other words, it's complicated. We're complicated. What works for us personally can be complicated, too.

You have something positive and helpful on your side when it comes to figuring out what works for you: *you*. Your body knows what works.

The exercises in this book are designed to help you better understand yourself. When a connection with your body is made, you can figure out for yourself if a change you try is working. Our bodies know what they need.

Byron Katie said, "Anything you want to ask a teacher, ask yourself and wait for the answer in silence." Start finding the answer to *Will this work for me?* by asking yourself. Sometimes the answer will be an outright *No!* Or maybe you'll get a nagging feeling that what you're doing isn't quite right. You're the specialist when it comes to your own body.

When we ask other specialists to help us as well, we add to the knowledge we gain by asking ourselves. That's what happened when I met with my allergist and discovered corn was the culprit.

The Right Combination

With MS, inflammation is the name of the game. Our immune systems are overachievers that cause problems in our central nervous systems. Most traditional drug therapies focus on lowering or changing the immune system in some way. When we get an infection, when we stress out, when we eat foods we're allergic to, it causes inflammation. Our immune systems get excited and work to try to cure us by reducing the inflammation.

But because we have MS, we don't want our immune systems to get excited. About anything. For us, an excited immune system is like a toddler helping you paint a wall: great intentions, big mess.

The issue of inflammation is a major reason why food is so important. When we figure out what foods cause inflammation in our bodies, we can stay away from them. But food reacts differently in different people's bodies. As you explore different foods and different combinations of foods, it's worthwhile to try to isolate your tests of individual food items. Pay attention to how your body feels so that you get specific results.

Seeking help from other specialists (besides yourself) can help you fine-tune your choices. Use different diets as guidelines, but continue to pay attention as you do so. Some aspects of a particular diet might work for you, but others might not, and you'll only know if you're asking your body for feedback and paying attention.

Food can help you heal, but only if it's the right food in the right combinations for you. The same goes for all the other areas that affect your MS and your life: what helps you is what's right for you. But there is a way to effectively track and work with all the different factors that affect us.

Shotguns Versus Layers

When we're looking for strategies that may help our MS stay under control, we often want to *do* something. We want someone who *knows* tell us what to do so we can take massive action. We can end up gathering tons of information from tons of different sources that have tons of different theories about what works. And most likely there are tons of contradictions as well, which create uncertainty around just what action we need to take. So what's a girl to do?

The shotgun approach, or trying a bunch of strategies at once, can seem like the answer. In theory, this approach may sound productive because we're making a lot of changes and taking things into our own hands. When we take tons of action like this the results can be scattered. This approach is not such a great tool for life-long changes that can help MS. This shotgun approach can lead to miscalculations about what is actually working and what is not.

Part of why I kept going back to a gluten-free diet when my body didn't feel right was because I had used the shotgun approach. I was trying so many different changes to my diet at the same time that I didn't know specifically which change was working and which wasn't. I couldn't see that a gluten-free diet wasn't the magic bullet for me, and so I missed out on finding the real culprit, corn, for a long time.

Trying everything at once to see what works doesn't allow much control over the results. You're likely to miss something or attribute a result to the wrong cause. Using this scattershot approach can feel frenzied, since it's all about fast action with little structure.

The approach I teach in my program is *layering*. Layering helps us make more meaningful changes, through tighter management, to provide a better understanding of what works. Try the things that make sense to you, but do it in a controlled environment so the results are clearer.

Layering allows you to create your own master plan for wellness.

For example, one layer of care may be reducing inflammation by changing your diet. Another layer may be optimizing sleep by focusing on getting enough hours of sleep a night. Another layer can be increased awareness of your thinking. Early on in our work together, I teach clients how to practice developing their thought awareness layer. Diet, sleep and awareness of what you're thinking are three distinct layers. Although ultimately everything works together, they're separate enough to observe changes. Make only one change in each layer at a time, so you can clearly see whether it helps you or not.

By making changes in these distinct layers, you can change more than one thing at a time while maintaining a clear focus on whether or not your new approach is working. For example, you can try out different ways of sleeping better, and quickly tell what's working and what's not. While you're going through that process, you can also add a layer of awareness about your thoughts. You may choose to develop the skill of letting go of unhelpful thoughts. At the same time, you can add a layer of physical activity, and start working out.

The key is to limit what you try to one change per layer so you don't run the risk of getting muddled feedback. You can experiment on multiple layers at the same time, trying lots of new ideas. When each layer is distinct enough, you have room to tweak it and thus really uncover what works for you, without your changes in another layer giving you a false result. There are fewer red herrings with this approach, because the results are specific to the layer being revised.

The layer approach is also valuable because good results within the layers will impact other layers positively. Discovering foods that work for your body will give you more energy for working out. Working out will help you sleep better. Sleeping well refreshes your willpower, so you're more motivated to keep exploring and thus discover even more of what works for you. And you'll have *thoughts* about working out, sleep, and diet changes, so you'll have plenty of opportunities to practice being aware of your thoughts.

Each layer changes your situation for the better. This layered approach gives you quality information about your individual body, and the layers work together to create an organic system tailored especially for you.

My Master Plan Discovery

I'm grateful to report that I am doing extremely well with my MS. People often ask me what I do to stay healthy, hoping I'll deliver a one-word solution they can start implementing immediately. I don't have a one-word answer, but I do have an answer: I stack the deck.

I layer multiple approaches and tweak them until they work for me. Each chapter of this book is about a layer I implement on a daily basis, and I'm consistently discovering new and different ways to optimize each layer.

As I said in the introduction, the chapters in this book are presented in the order I discovered each layer, except for the diet layer, which I've worked on since I was diagnosed. At first, I used the shotgun method with my diet, but it wasn't until I became more systematic about my layers that I found which foods work best for me. And each layer positively influenced the next.

After my diagnosis, I began working out. That led me to noticing that what I *thought* about exercise determined whether or not I put on my running shoes. As I became more aware of my thoughts, I noticed that I was numb emotionally and needed to do some work to understand how I felt. I then noticed that I felt stressed all the time, so I started trying to bring down my stress levels by understanding the correlation between my stress and my thoughts. That created deeper awareness of my own thoughts, and I became very aware of how hard I was being on myself and that I was severely lacking in self-love. When I became kinder to myself, a spark was lit and I noticed that it was possible to do even more to cultivate my energy. When all of those layers came into play, I felt much more in control of my body, my MS, and more, and that allowed me to be completely honest with myself about my fears and denials.

These chapters represent some of the main layers that I've implemented, but there are many more layers that can be added, such as weight loss, social connections, and boundaries.

A layer I've had in place from the day I was diagnosed was some form of traditional drug therapy. I don't discuss it much in this book, because I believe the choice to use drug therapy or not is between you and your doctor. Even though I work very closely with my MS specialist and trust him completely, I still consult my body about whether or not the medication works. I've been through multiple medications. Some have worked better than others, and some didn't work at all. Connecting with my body has been crucial to navigating the decision-making process about which medications were worth staying with and which ones weren't for me after all.

I won't do anything long-term based solely on someone else's opinion that it's good to do. Taking medication is no exception.

Try It—Develop Your Master Plan

Optimizing your layering takes practice, especially when you're beginning to pay attention to these things for the first time. When I practiced each of the layers I present in this book, I went about it like I'd learn any other new skill: try, fail, and try again.

You may already have some layers in place. Write down each layer and note what you're currently doing that you know works. For example, one layer may be sleep. What you're currently doing that works for you may include going to bed each night at a certain time, or with a specific temperature setting for the room you sleep in. I suggest using a separate sheet of paper or the worksheet at the end of this section to track each layer.

The first step of this exercise is to identify what's currently working—not what you've done in the past or what you want to try next (that comes later). This is an inventory of what you're doing right now. This inventory is important to have, not only as a base to build upon, but because we tend to be doing way more to help ourselves than we give ourselves credit for.

At the top of each sheet, write down the name of the layer and your personal reason for implementing that layer. Your personal reason is your *why*, as discussed in Chapter 2, that's important for keeping your motivation and drive strong for each layer.

Now look over your layers. Is there an existing layer you would like to develop further? Is there a new layer you would like to start?

For example, if exercise is an existing layer you'd like to develop further, write down information about what's currently going on. Do you currently have a workout that you like? How often do you do it? What do you do during each workout? How would you like to develop this layer further? Do you want to try something different? Do you want to increase or decrease the frequency?

List one thing you want to do toward developing this layer. To continue the exercise example, you could increase your cardio time by five minutes or add two new stretches at the end of the workout. Start with little changes. You're creating new personal habits, which is no small task. If you make the change too big or too fast, it will have a lesser chance of sticking.

Focus on that one new layer for one month. Take notes about what works and what doesn't, and try the next changes only after you've gotten answers about the previous change you tried.

Developing a master plan may look like adding layers to try something new, but it also may look like subtracting layers by removing something you're currently doing. For example, maybe you discover you're working out too much and need to cut back to one day a week to feel even better. This is still developing a layer.

After one month, start developing your next layer.

Maybe the next layer is brand new. Choose it by noticing what new layer resonates with you as something you'd like to find out about. What have you wanted to try?

Approach subsequent layers the same way as described above. If you're not currently doing anything in a particular in a layer, you can ask yourself what you want to try next. When you add a layer to try out a change, that layer should be totally different from the other layers you're currently working to adjust. For example, if your first layer was exercise, you may want to try thought awareness next.

Write down one small step to try in this new layer. An example could be doing one Thought Storm worksheet every day, if you're working on the thought awareness layer. Focus on this layer for one month, noting what works and what doesn't.

As you add each layer, the previous layers remain in place. You may need to tweak the existing layers a bit as time goes on, but try to maintain an awareness of the current status of each layer in your master plan.

Build these layers slowly and methodically, by keeping track of what you do. Remember to write down the reason you're doing the specific activities in each layer. You may feel like it takes a while to build up the layers in a way that makes an overall impact. Don't worry—what you're doing has an impact and you will have multiple layers within months. You'll start to notice a difference sooner than you think.

My Master Plan

....

Layer: _____

Why is this important to you? _____
_____
_____
_____

Current techniques used: _____
_____
_____
_____

How can I make this better? _____
_____
_____
_____

New techniques I want to try: _____
_____
_____
_____

Notes: _____
_____
_____
_____
_____

START CREATING YOUR OWN MASTER PLAN.
Go to *www.AndreaHansonCoaching.com/BookSheets*
and download your free worksheets.

This Is Not a Straight Line

In this book, I tell you how I tried one thing that led to another and another and how that has helped. As you do this for yourself, you may realize what I realized—that nothing about this process is tidy. Refocusing on one layer may allow you to optimize a layer you'd thought was already running smoothly enough. Then focusing on different layer may make you question whether you're doing the right thing at all, with either layer, because those two layers are impacting each other in a way that's not feeling so great. That's ok. Second-guessing and changing your mind and getting frustrated can all, ultimately, be productive parts of this process.

There may be days when sitting on the sofa and consuming delicious cheesy poofs and reality TV are part of the process, too. Those days may happen when you're making progress and being pushed out of your comfort zone. My master plan will always be evolving. Sometimes chocolate is part of that evolution.

It's ok if you try something that backfires. That's another piece of knowledge gained that you didn't have before. Don't let fear keep you from trying something new. Even if you're scared, you can go ahead. Find your courage and try it anyway. Don't let getting frustrated discourage you, because you may find that on the other side of the frustration is a discovery that was worth the journey.

Most importantly, don't let failure convince you that someone else knows better than you about what you should do.

What layers will you start with to move your master plan forward? What area or areas in your life most need optimizing? Those are great places to begin.

Creating a master plan that keeps you feeling good on all the layers will likely not happen by moving in a straight line. Allow yourself to find progress by going back and forth, and side to side, but keep learning as you go. Your growth may pull you up and down. Keep going. Trust that your mind and body have the answers. Be patient, courageous, and, most importantly, compassionate with yourself as you figure out what works for you for managing your MS.

Yes, it can be done.

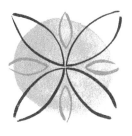

········

Chapter 10

········

Moving Forward

You didn't ask for MS. You don't want it. And you certainly didn't do anything to deserve it. You really just want to go home. Home is where you're safe. Home is where nothing can get to you. Home is where you can relax and get away from all the stress and anxiety of life. Home is where your "normal" life is.

I understand feeling exhausted thinking about everything there is to do. Searching Google for answers and then, once you find them, not knowing if those answers are going to be valid for you, your body, and your unique situation. I understand wanting MS and everything that comes with it to go away so you don't have to deal with the changes.

I understand that having MS can feel hard.

But you have options.

Courage

Getting ahead of your MS is a new skill to master. It takes courage to look at something scary and get know it intimately enough to understand how it works and what calms it down.

Don't sell yourself short.

You *do* have that courage. By reading this book, you've already proven your willingness to look inside. You've already shown yourself that you can take a look at something you'd rather not look at and learn more about it.

Moving forward with courage can be daunting. Courage can feel uncomfortable in our bodies. It's the feeling that often shows up when we're launching ourselves into something big and unknown. But courage isn't an all or nothing proposition. It can start in small bits, in little movements. Your job is to recognize your courage every time it shows up. No matter how small or fleeting, own it every time you feel courage rise up. Little by little, that courage will evolve from a hint into an impressive force.

Connection

I wish I could make our MS go away. I would pay big money for the magic wand that could do that. Although there are hundreds of millions of dollars going into MS research, we don't have a cure—yet. There are impressive disease-modifying therapies currently being researched, and I do believe we will see a cure in our lifetimes. Until then, the best method we have to reduce the effects of MS is to be the healthiest humans possible.

That approach is *not* one-size-fits-all.

It's up to us each, individually, to connect with ourselves and discover what will work for us. Even the best doctors in the world can't tell us how we feel. We need to stay connected to ourselves, be mindful about what we think and believe, and stay tuned in to how we feel emotionally. We need to listen to our bodies. And honor what they tell us.

The good news is that we don't need anything other than what we already have right now in order to improve our health. Exercise doesn't have to take place in a gym that charges membership fees. We can go outside, or even stay in our own homes, and still get a great workout. Diet doesn't have to include pricey foods. In fact, learning to cook with whole foods can be more satisfying and easier on the budget than eating prepared meals or eating out. Thoughts, emotions, energy, stress, kindness, and honesty are all free. In fact, they're all here now, waiting for us to pay attention. I promise that connecting with yourself is not too mysterious a process to figure out and benefit from.

Every single one of us carries a backpack that fills with bricks as life goes on. Each brick represents a circumstance in our life. Some people are aware of their backpack and the bricks inside and some people aren't. The people who are aware can manage and carry their backpacks more skillfully and may even figure out ways to lighten their load. But the backpack, however full, doesn't weigh them down.

Your backpack doesn't have to weigh you down, either.

As you create a stronger connection with yourself, your connections with others will change as well. Your current relationships will become more compelling and you'll create new relationships. Friends, family, and professionals will seem to come out of thin air and be exactly what you need at just the right time. We are all in this life together. It's amazing to discover how many people will want to help you, just as you would want to help them.

Life is a journey that doesn't have to be traveled alone.

Trust

You're facing big changes. You may not know when these unwanted changes will slow down or stop. You may have lots of doctors and advice and support, but ultimately there's one big thing you'll need in order to get through this.

You need to trust in yourself.

Trusting myself was a tough layer to add, but once I started working on it I saw how essential it is. We're making a lot of decisions as we deal with our MS. Sometimes the results of our decisions aren't immediately evident and so we have to trust that our decisions are right.

What we expect to happen is extremely important in determining outcomes. And expectations don't live long without trust.

Trust sometimes has bad associations, like that it's hard to get and harder to keep. Trust has to be earned. Trustworthiness has to be demonstrated before trust is given. And trust can be broken if promises aren't delivered.

We're tough on trust and easy on doubt. But doubt doesn't serve us when we want to create a stronger connection with ourselves. Doubt keeps us from truly forming that bond, because it makes us second-guess whether we know what's best. And doubting ourselves slows us down when we have to make decisions. We're less stressed and make better progress when we trust that we're doing what's best for ourselves, always, even if we later need to make changes and go in a different direction. We trust ourselves to know what is needed, and trust ourselves to make a new choice.

I'm not talking about trusting a stranger you just met. This is you. Your inner connection may feel new as you try new things, but you already know so much about yourself. As you move forward with decisions, notice whether your full trust is present. If it's not, ask yourself why. That answer can reveal a belief you're holding that needs uncovering and releasing. Keep moving toward an unwavering confidence, and trust that you can figure out what's best for you.

The Bottom Line

MS doesn't have to rule your life. Even the symptoms of MS don't have to rule your life. I've worked with people with major disabilities who feel 100 percent in control of their well-being. I've also worked with people who have next to no symptoms who live every day in fear of what their MS will do to them.

It's how you look at your MS that creates your reactions. Changing the way you think about MS has the power to change your life for the better in big ways. How you feel inside, how you take care of yourself, the mood you're in when you wake up each morning, these are all influenced by what you make it mean to have MS.

Do you make having MS mean you're fragile and have to change everything you love about your life? Do you make it mean that the future is frightening and unknown? Or do you make having MS mean that even though you have an extra brick in your backpack, you know what it is and you will keep moving forward?

I asked you a question in Chapter 1. Hopefully you've been redefining your answer as you read through the book and tried the meditations and exercises. Now I'll ask you that crucial question again: *Who do you want to be as a person living with MS?*

Who you *want* to be as a person living with MS can also be who you *expect* to be.

Trust that you will do everything in your power to make your expectation a reality.

Thoughts to Leave You With

You are in charge.

Always.

Not your doctors. Not your parents.

Not your partners or your kids or your ex-whatever.

And certainly not your MS.

You *are*.
Without question.
How do you want to feel right now?
How do you want to feel about your MS?

Whatever your answer, it's possible.
You can make this journey mean whatever you want.
Good or bad.
Success or failure.
Living free or living in a cage.

Only you can do it.
In fact, only you must do it.
And, yes, you are strong enough.

I won't lie to you—this can be tough.
But so are you.
There will be bumps. But you can ride them all.
There will be fears. But you can be afraid and move forward anyway.

Hold on to your control.
Hold on to your love and support for yourself.
Hold on to what's working and what you can make even better in the future.
Most importantly, hold onto you.

Because even through the tears and the mistakes,
through your best sit-down-and-sulk protests, you are enough.

You're the strongest ally you will have.
You.
A force to be reckoned with.

Acknowledgments

....

There is an inner circle of people without whom this book would not exist. I owe more than I can put on the page to them—for their expertise, love, encouragement, and hard work—and their generosity for sharing it with me.

To Claude Paul, for telling me it's all going to be ok when I forget. I love you more than anything. To Dr. F. for all the advice, knowledge, and support you've given me for 15 years and counting. You were the first to tell me I should write this book, and I'm grateful you planted that seed. To Teresa, for being a foundation for my sanity and my health. I'm not sure you know just how often you've calmed my inner gremlins. To Cinzia, for showing me the fears in my head and helping me trust my heart. Your encouragement means everything. To my family for (mostly) not laughing when I told you about this crazy dream of mine five years ago. I love every one of you. To Mom and my big sister Kerry, for your unconditional support. I wouldn't be here without you. To Grace, for saving my bacon more times than I can count. Writing is an incredibly vulnerable and humbling process, and I'm so glad I went through it with you. This book would, literally, not be here without you. To my clients, thank you for making this an easy path to choose. Your strength is inspiring.

To Dad, for sitting on my hospital bed that night and giving me permission to keep moving forward. You told me exactly what I needed to hear and I will never forget those words.

About the Author

....

Andrea Wildenthal Hanson was diagnosed with multiple sclerosis in 2000. Since then she's learned that the key to managing this disease is not being an expert in MS—it's being an expert in *you*. Andrea combines her experience from five years of life and weight loss coaching and 17-plus years of living with MS to provide clients with a customized approach to living well with a chronic illness.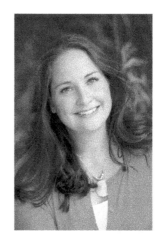

She received her bachelor's degree in Psychology at the University of North Texas, and her master's degree in Human Development with a specialty in Early Childhood Disorders from the University of Texas at Dallas. Andrea then became a Certified Life Coach at Martha Beck Inc., a Certified Weight Loss Coach and a Master Certified Coach at the Life Coach School.

As well as running her own coaching business, Andrea worked with the National MS Society as a coach for their Planning Wise employment program and the Every Day Matters program teaching positive thinking. The Summer 2014 issue of *MS Connections* magazine featured and interview with Andrea on her work with helping people with MS stay employed. She has run classes for the MAPSS-MS (Memory, Attention and Problem Solving Skills for Persons with MS) research team at the University of Texas at Austin.

When she's not traveling, she lives in the Colorado Rockies with her husband, Clay, and their perfect dog, Budd Friday.

Thank You Gift

EXCLUSIVE OFFER FOR READERS OF
LIVE YOUR LIFE, NOT YOUR DIAGNOSIS:
Receive a special gift at no additional cost
when you download your free companion worksheets.
To find out more, *visit*
www.AndreaHansonCoaching.com/BookSheets.

FOR MORE FROM ANDREA W HANSON,
LISTEN TO HER FREE PODCAST:
The Health Mindset Podcast
www.AndreaHansonCoaching.com

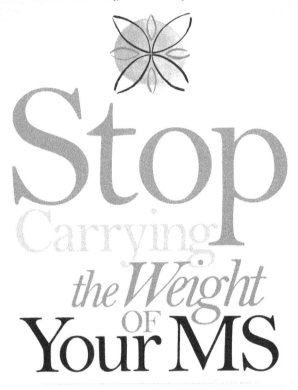

foreword by

ALEXA STUIFBERGEN, PhD, RN, FAAN

Dean, James Dougherty Centennial
Professor of Nursing, The University of Texas at Austin

Stop Carrying

the Weight

OF

Your MS

The Art of *Losing Weight,*

Healing Your Body, and

Soothing Your Multiple Sclerosis

Andrea Wildenthal Hanson

Stop Carrying the Weight of Your MS

Chapter 1

....

Important Questions

Abby was diagnosed with multiple sclerosis five years ago. Like many people facing a diagnosis, she was shocked when she heard the news. In her eyes, too much testing and time went by before she got the diagnosis. But at least, finally, she had an answer to what was happening to her.

Before her diagnosis, her legs kept tingling and feeling like pins and needles. She went to the doctor each time it happened, but was told that being overweight was most likely compressing a nerve in her back. The pins and needles would go away periodically, and so she thought she was fine.

Until she wasn't.

Now she has an explanation for what's going on with her health and has done her research on MS. She's lucky to have a good neurologist and drug treatment options. She knows—for the most part—what's happening with her body. She also knows that there's a lot she can do on her own to help her prognosis with this disease.

Abby is smart and can be categorized as an overachiever, although she just sees it as getting stuff done. She's the go-to for everything at her job and in her family. She likes it that way. Even though sometimes she wishes people would figure it out themselves, she's glad to be the "fixer."

Abby is doing well at work and sees promotion in her future. In fact, she sees a lot in her future—family, travel, adventures. What she never saw in her future was disability, illness, and hospital bills. When she's being totally honest with herself, a future involving any kind of dependency scares the hell out of her. *What if MS wrecks my life?*

Right now, she's doing well enough. The pins and needles in her legs are still there, but she can handle that. Other symptoms, like optic neuritis, have come and gone, but she gets steroids each time and recovers. She's strong, and she relies on that strength every day. But she can't help wondering, *if I'm so strong that I can have this great career, support my family and go out with friends, then why am I not strong enough to lose this extra weight?*

She tells herself that she should have this weight thing figured out by now.

It has occurred to her that she might have been accurately diagnosed with MS years earlier if she had been at a healthier body weight. *If the doctor didn't have weight to blame, would he have considered testing for MS sooner?* That's a question she knows will never be answered. But her motive still stands: if she wants to have that future without being dependent on someone else, she knows she needs to be as healthy as possible, starting now.

And she knows that means losing weight.

She was overweight before her diagnosis, so this isn't a new issue for her. But since then she's put on even more weight. Some of the weight is definitely from the steroids. *Those things are evil*, she tells herself. But she knows the steroids aren't the only things to blame for her weight. There isn't good food at the office, and her husband keeps junk food well-stocked in the kitchen at home. She feels sabotaged every time she turns around, and then there's the added pressure of MS on top of it.

I have to get on top of this, she tells herself.

Now that MS is in play, Abby is even more motivated to lose weight—and to do it the "right" way. She wants to exercise, but she doesn't love her options. She knows she wants to clean up her diet, but is unclear on the best things to eat (and not eat) for a person who has MS. She doesn't want to simply jump into something, and she knows she can lose weight and help her MS at the same time—*but how?*

She gets online to try and figure it out. There is no shortage of direct instructions in her research. She finds countless nutritionists, dieticians, doctors, and naturopaths that tell her exactly what to eat and what to avoid. The problem is they all say different things. *Who are these people?* She asks herself. *Are they any good? Does this diet really work?* As she explores, she finds testimonials for every diet that say not only that it works, but that it works fast.

If she combines all these diets and does everything these people say is essential for MS, she'll be able to eat exactly… *nothing*. She knows for a fact she doesn't want to be one of *those people*. She cringes when she thinks about not being able to go out to eat any more. She cringes even more when she thinks about taking ten minutes to order a salad because she has to explain her very important list of what she can't have to the waiter (a list she's pretty sure will be ignored, anyway).

One thing Abby has heard a lot about in her research about good diets for people with MS is going gluten-free. *Everyone with an autoimmune disease is doing this. I'm sure it will make me feel better and lose weight*, she thinks to herself. So she cuts out gluten to see if that helps. She's been doing it really diligently for two weeks now, but she has no idea if it's working. She has no idea because when she stepped on the scale this morning, she saw that she had gained back the two pounds she lost last week.

How can other people do this so easily? What's wrong with me?

She sighs and checks her Instagram feed for a mental break. This research hurts her head. She just wants to think about something else for a while.

Within five minutes, she sees an ad on Instagram about gut flora being the key to everything. A post about how avocados can cure MS shows up as she scrolls. She sighs again. *This isn't helping.* She's already avoiding her personal messages because a friend forwarded her an article. "Thought of you!" the message said, and her friend attached a study about spinach possibly being bad for people with MS. Abby knows her friend means well but she also knows her friend didn't actually read the article before sharing it. Abby forgives her for sending something based on just the reading of a headline, but she doesn't have the energy or time right now to read another word about what she can't have.

She closes her laptop and just sits there. Frustrated, confused, annoyed. Her neurologist hasn't really helped beyond telling her that losing weight will help her MS and to eat less and move more.

She feels like a failure as she asks herself (for the thousandth time), *Why can't I figure this out?*

Feeling like she's failing is so foreign to Abby. Everyone who knows her would say she's a positive person. She believes that attitude is everything. She works very hard to see the positive in every person and situation. She starts to worry that maybe her weight is the exception to that rule.

Shaking it off, she decides that she's done with searching for the answer for now. *I have work to do. I don't have time for this now.* She welcomes the distraction of getting her files put back in her bag for work in the morning. She goes to sleep trying to be positive. Trying to believe the answer will come to her. Trying to be strong. And yet still worried that, if she can't figure out this weight thing, her future may look very different than she hopes.

Oh #@*%, the harsh reality hits her, *where I want to go in my life may not ever happen if I don't figure this out.*

The Missing Piece

Abby feels bounced around while she searches for an answer. As she starts to do one thing, she finds another expert saying to do something completely different. It's a rollercoaster ride she wishes would stop.

Finding your own answers can be just as frustrating. It's like standing in line at the DMV for hours, only to be told at the window that you were in the wrong line and need to start over. Then you beat yourself up for not reading the signs more carefully. It can make giving yourself breaks from focusing on weight loss seem like the kind thing to do.

There's a reason for this constant disappointment. Frustration often emerges when we're lacking in one very key element: confidence. When we're confident that we know what we're doing, we're not so insecure about being "right." You're confident you can read the words on this page. If a group of people told you that you were reading this wrong, their words wouldn't make you stop and wonder how to do it right. You probably wouldn't mind them at all. Because you're confident that you're reading this the right way.

It can be difficult to find that confidence when we keep thinking that others know better than we do. It makes sense that we feel inferior when we continue to ask other people how to make us healthy instead of asking ourselves.

How can you be assured that something is working if you don't ask the only person with firsthand knowledge about your body?

Consulted instead are the doctors, nutritionists, the internet, and the scale. You defer to experiences of other people when really you need to trust your own body.

What if we knew more about our own bodies than the experts?

How differently would you approach new information and advice? What would you think about the tiny study saying spinach is bad when you just had a spinach salad and knew you feel great? If you had that confidence—the confidence that you were the expert about your own body—you wouldn't be as likely to let bits of random information push you around into questionable territory.

But sometimes having confidence feels even more out of reach than losing weight. You may ask yourself, *How can I have confidence when nothing I do seems to be working?*

The One Thing We Know for Sure

Right now you may be as frustrated and annoyed as Abby. You may simply want to know how to lose weight. You may want someone to just *tell* you what to do.

The one thing you *can* know for sure is you are exactly where you need to be. I completely understand how ridiculous that sounds. When I was crying alone in my apartment because I'd only allowed myself to eat one grape for dessert, I would have smacked myself for saying that. But here's the thing—if I had been okay with that very restrictive diet, I would have stayed there. I would still be on it—if I didn't want more for myself (literally and figuratively). But I knew that beating myself up over one grape wasn't the answer, so I searched for more. I had the desire to find a better plan that worked for my weight loss, and for my MS. Stressing myself out over what to eat wasn't the right plan for me.

Sometimes desire looks like frustration, annoyance, even trepidation, and that's exactly where you need to be to find a better path.

Your desire has led you here, looking for a weight loss plan that works for you. You're now diving into the main source of knowledge that holds the key to being healthy: *you.*

You may not feel qualified to take that big step into the role of expert just yet, and that's okay. Small, slow steps are all you need to take your rightful place of being the authority on your health. This book is a map of steps to help you get the traction you need so your doctor visits no longer have that element of *I have to lose the weight* shame. Most importantly, you'll gain the confidence to know that your future with MS is bright and full of the adventure you crave.

Starting off, you may be a bit skeptical.

If you're like I was when I looked for the answers, you have little trust in yourself about losing weight. You may be looking back at how your weight loss has gone in the past and finding all sorts of evidence that you don't know how to do it. Or, what can feel worse, you may have proven to yourself that you *do* know what will help, but you don't have the discipline to stick with it. You may think the bottom line is what the scale says, and the scale is not being very kind to you.

These are all perfectly normal ways to feel about weight loss. We put ourselves under a lot of pressure to figure it out.

Let's Go

I was a lot like Abby. I was diagnosed with MS in 2000. I was overweight and the multiple rounds of steroids didn't help. I already had plenty of body shame around how much I weighed and, after the diagnosis, the fresh shame of having MS sat like a cherry on top. I wasn't stupid—I knew that what I ate and my lifestyle of stress and partying was abusing my body. I secretly feared that all the abuse led me to develop MS—and that everyone else was secretly thinking that, too.

When I reached the end of my rope, I looked for the answers outside of myself. Probably much like you, I wasn't happy with the answers I got. They weren't resonating with me. Whenever I followed diet advice or lifestyle recommendations, I felt like I was wearing the wrong size shoe. It looked pretty, and I wanted so badly for it to fit, but it just didn't. And that left me feeling lacking and depleted.

I did eventually find the right people who showed me the way. But they weren't diet experts, or even doctors. They were teachers, philosophers, and poets. They were the ones who told me I'd been the expert all along. They showed me how to make peace with my body and listen to it. They showed me how to tap into my own body's genius and use it to heal myself.

Just like I will show you how to heal yourself, too.

I will never have everything all figured out, and neither will you. I fully expect to have serious (organic, free range) potato chip cravings as I write this book. And that's just fine. Because the difference in me now is that I have the confidence to know that, when I do start to backslide, I can pull myself out of it way faster—and without all the heartache. I now understand how to listen to expert advice while staying true to myself—something that continues to help me discover which foods make my body sing and which don't. I'll teach you the tools that taught me what lifestyle makes my body fat melt away—so that you can find what works like that for you. I'll also show you tools I use to find that sweet spot of working out that keeps me feeling strong and vibrant—and how to adjust as I change.

The most important change is that I stopped feeling like a pinball being thrown around, thinking maybe this next person will know better than I do. I know that other people may have data that's useful, but I am the only one who has the right answer for me.

It's your time to become that person for yourself.

I understand this may feel big. It *is* big. But it doesn't have to be *scary*, and you're not doing this alone.

In these pages, I'm here as your coach, helping you through your path to finally finding the real answers. I'm not only going to show you the steps to take, but also help you with the internal struggles that may come when you take action. I'll be there with you for the doubts and the fears and will show you how to get around them and get back on course.

Not everyone with MS is seeking a solution like you are. Some are content to wait for directions on what to do. Others find more fulfillment in restating the problem than finding the solution. What you're doing takes courage. Wear that badge of honor while you go through this book, knowing that acting on your desire to get in control of your life and your MS symptoms sets you apart.

Allow me to hold your hand and answer your questions. Allow me to ask you the important questions to answer for yourself. You can do this. You were born to take control. I have no doubt.

Let's go.

WHY IS WEIGHT LOSS SO CONFUSING— ESPECIALLY WHEN YOU HAVE A DIAGNOSIS?

Listen to the free downloadable audio from me
to get the answers to:

- What exactly is standing in my way?
- What's the real reason why traditional dieting only works for a short time?
- How can I make weight loss stick for good?

For your instant download, visit:
www.AndreaHansonCoaching.com/Learnmore.

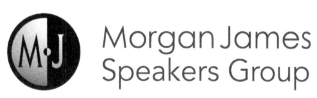

Morgan James
Speakers Group

www.TheMorganJamesSpeakersGroup.com

We connect Morgan James published authors with live and online events and audiences who will benefit from their expertise.

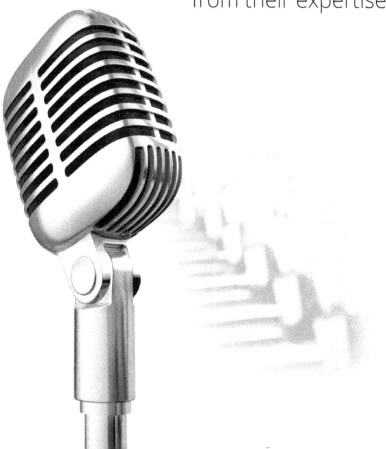

Printed in the USA
CPSIA information can be obtained
at www.ICGtesting.com
JSHW082341140824
68134JS00020B/1807